YOUR POWER TO HEAL

Incredible Natural Ways to Manage
Your Weight, Fight Diabetes,
Relieve Arthritis Pain, Lower
Your Blood Pressure, and More!

Publisher's Note

This book is intended for general information only. It does not constitute medical, legal, or financial advice or practice. The editors of FC&A have taken careful measures to ensure the accuracy and usefulness of the information in this book. While every attempt has been made to assure accuracy, errors may occur. Some websites, addresses, and telephone numbers may have changed since printing. We cannot guarantee the safety or effectiveness of any advice or treatments mentioned. Readers are urged to consult with their professional financial advisors, lawyers, and health care professionals before making any changes.

Any health information in this book is for information only and is not intended to be a medical guide for self-treatment. It does not constitute medical advice and should not be construed as such or used in place of your doctor's medical advice. Readers are urged to consult with their health care professionals before undertaking therapies suggested by the information in this book, keeping in mind that errors in the text may occur as in all publications and that new findings may supersede older information.

The publisher and editors disclaim all liability (including any injuries, damages, or losses) resulting from the use of the information in this book.

> *"He gives strength to the weary, and to him who lacks might He increases power."*
>
> *Isaiah 40:29*

FC&A Medical Publishing®
103 Clover Green
Peachtree City, GA 30269

Produced by the staff of FC&A

ISBN 978-1935574804

Contents

Contents

Contents

Contents

Contents

Allergies

Easy natural relief

Allergies have become the sixth-leading cause of disease in the United States, affecting more than 50 million Americans and costing the health care system more than $18 billion a year.

You can be allergic to almost anything, with reactions ranging from a slightly stuffy nose to life-threatening anaphylactic shock. The most common allergy is allergic rhinitis or hay fever. Some scientists think better health and hygiene are partly responsible for rising allergies. It could be that children who are kept away from germs have less chance to build up an immunity to viruses.

Drugstore shelves are full of prescription and over-the-counter (OTC) remedies, so it's easy to spend a lot of money searching for allergy relief. Here are some things you can do to make yourself feel better without breaking the bank.

Secret to cheap prevention

One of the least expensive things you can do to allergy-proof your home is to clean it often and well. Among the allergens you need to eliminate inside your house are dust mites, mold, animal dander, and cockroach droppings.

Clean your air with ivy. New research shows English ivy can wipe out airborne allergens from things like mold spores and animal feces.

Target dust mites. Get rid of the allergy-causing residue from microscopic pests by dusting surfaces and washing bed linens in hot water at least once a week. Launder blankets and mattress pads four times a year.

Keep humidity low. Dust mites, mold, and mildew thrive in a damp environment, so keep humidity levels below 40 percent, and don't let moisture build up in the kitchen and bathroom. You can use mold-killing cleansers in sinks, showers, and tubs. A study partially funded by The Clorox Company found that diluted household bleach not only kills mold but also neutralizes mold allergens.

Vacuum frequently. Most experts recommend vacuuming once or twice a week. But some say it's not effective at removing dust mites, even with the use of expensive filter bags. Although vacuuming sweeps up some allergens, it also stirs up dust in the air. It's best to wear a mask when doing housework or have someone who isn't allergic do it. Better yet, replace carpets with hard surfaces, and confine pets to areas where you don't spend a lot of time.

Keep pests from coming back. You may need an exterminator to get rid of cockroaches, mice, and other pests. But that's only half the battle. The allergens come from their body residue and droppings, so you need to clean your house thoroughly after the exterminator is finished. Discourage the return of these pests by cutting out food and water sources. Don't leave dirty dishes in the sink, and clean up spills and crumbs immediately.

Fight to get the right medicine

Your health insurance may no longer pay for the allergy medicine that works best for you. Since Claritin is now available without a prescription and as a generic, insurance companies are raising deductibles or refusing to pay at all for prescription antihistamines.

But the substitute drugs don't always work as well for some people. If that's the case for you, talk to your doctor about convincing the insurance company you need a particular medicine. He can submit a "prior authorization" form to your insurer saying the drug they'll pay for doesn't work for you. Then you can ask the company to cover the drug you like.

Another solution is to talk to your doctor about using nasal corticosteroids instead of antihistamines. Nasonex and Rhinocort, for example, don't have as many restrictions as Allegra and Zyrtec. For many people, the steroids also seem to be more effective.

Shut down sneezing with allergy shots

Allergen immunotherapy can be a successful solution to your sniffing and sneezing when all else fails. You need to see an allergy specialist, who will run tests to find out exactly what you are allergic to. Then the allergist will inject you with increasing amounts of those allergens over a period of several months.

The shots work like a vaccine and, after a while, you build up an immunity to the allergens. The American Academy of Allergy, Asthma & Immunology (AAAAI) says this treatment is successful in up to 90 percent of patients with seasonal allergic rhinitis.

Allergy shots are a drastic measure because of the time, trouble, and expense they involve. But they could be worth it, depending on the extent of your allergy problem and whether you can control it with drugs. You'll eventually make up the cost from the money you save on allergy medicine.

To find a certified allergist/immunologist in your area, call the AAAAI at 414-272-6071 or go to *www.aaaai.org* on the Internet. You can also use the American College of Allergy, Asthma & Immunology at *www.acaai.org*.

Best way to breathe allergen-free air

Pollens, molds, and animal dander can float around inside your house as well as outside. If you sneeze even when you're indoors, an air cleaner may be what you need to keep allergens from bothering you. Here are some things to consider before you buy.

▸ Air filtration alone is not a solution for reducing indoor allergens. You also need to control sources of pollution, have adequate ventilation, and keep surfaces clean where allergens come to rest.

▸ The Clean Air Delivery Rate (CADR) for tobacco smoke should be at least two-thirds your room's area in square feet. For a 10'x12' room (120 sq. ft.), you need a machine with a CADR of 80.

▸ Not all air purifiers actually filter particles out of the air. Some are intended to kill bacteria or eliminate odors and gases. See the chart on the following page for the different ways air cleaners work.

Air cleaner	How it works	Pros and cons
Mechanical filter	Air is forced through a mesh that traps particles of pollen, tobacco smoke, pet dander, and other irritants.	HEPA (high efficiency particulate air) filters catch pollutants .03 microns or larger. ULPA filters catch even smaller parts.
Electronic or ionization filter	Static electricity causes particles to stick to the filter.	Some units may create ozone above an acceptable level.
Ozone generator	Uses ozone to oxidize organic compounds that produce odors.	Has little effect on allergens. Creates ozone above acceptable levels.

Save money with natural antihistamines

Histamines are naturally occurring chemicals that cause allergic reactions in your body. It shouldn't be surprising, then, to know that naturally occurring antihistamines might counteract those reactions. Try these naturals instead of expensive allergy medicines.

Vitamin C is perhaps nature's best-known solution for allergies. It seems to keep your white blood cells from releasing histamines and then neutralizes the ones that do appear. Research shows your histamine levels rise when you don't get enough C, so eat peppers, citrus fruits, and other foods rich in vitamin C regularly. It works best when you get it all the time, not just when your allergies flare up.

Quercetin is another food chemical that regulates histamine release, and you'll find plenty in apples and onions. Quercetin is even more effective when combined with bromelain, an anti-inflammatory agent found in pineapple. Bromelain boosts quercetin's absorption.

Herbal supplements may be the answer if you don't get enough of these nutrients from foods. Other herbal aids for allergies include freeze-dried stinging nettle and butterbur extract, which are only available as supplements. Talk to your doctor before you take extra pills, though. If you take other allergy drugs along with the naturals, you can get in trouble from too much antihistamine activity.

Sweet way to ease symptoms

Here's an oh-so-sweet way to ease allergy symptoms without using drugs — if it really works.

Some people swear by the powers of local honey to build up your immune system so you won't be bothered by the sniffing, sneezing, and itchy eyes of hay fever. It has to be made by bees that gather pollen in the area where you live, and it has to be unfiltered. The idea is that your body won't react to pollen in the honey because it comes into your body through your digestive system. After a while, your immune system also stops reacting to the pollen when you breathe it in.

For whatever reason, people say it works. But research to back it up is hard to find. If you love honey, it may be worth a try to find a local beekeeper and start eating the honey before allergy season begins. But be careful — it's also possible to be allergic to honey. Doctors aren't sure if it's because of the pollen or for some other reason, but if you notice any unusual symptoms, stop taking it.

Beware of money-wasting therapies

Homeopathy has a lot in common with local honey as a cure for allergies. It's based on the idea that the same substance that causes a disease can also cure it, but there is no clear scientific evidence it actually works.

Homeopathic allergy medicine is just a highly diluted form of a specific allergen, so you can't be sure exactly what is in the bottle. Active ingredients are repeatedly diluted, so the medicine may contain only water or alcohol and won't cause any harm. But, in some cases,

Exciting allergy cures on the horizon

You may soon be able to block pollen with a simple nose cream. A German company has come up with an ointment that traps pollen before it can cause trouble for your allergies. A study paid for by the manufacturer found the cream cut allergic symptoms by nearly 60 percent with no adverse effects.

A Swiss vaccine company is experimenting with a DNA-based dust-mite vaccine they say reduces hay fever symptoms. It is also working on vaccines against cat hair as well as grass and tree pollen. In Japan, an edible vaccine made from genetically modified rice also shows promise. It has been shown to cut allergy symptoms in mice.

products are diluted only a little and may contain significant amounts of the active ingredient. This can lead to problems with side effects.

Acupuncture is another complementary-alternative medicine (CAM) used to treat allergies. Like homeopathy, scientists have trouble proving acupuncture and other CAMs are effective. They urge caution when using alternative remedies because of their high cost and potential risks, such as dangerous side effects.

Alternative remedies may work like a placebo in some cases, but most people are better off saving their money for proven allergy remedies.

Shun foods that affect your seasonal allergies

One in three people with seasonal allergies also have oral allergy syndrome. Their immune systems confuse the proteins in certain foods with the proteins in pollen, triggering an attack. You could be one of them if you develop sniffles, sneezes, or an itchy mouth, lips, or throat after eating certain raw or fresh fruits and other foods.

Most reactions are minor and harmless, says allergist Joseph Leija. But if you develop trouble breathing or an itchy rash, he advises you go to a board-certified allergist or, in extreme cases, straight to the emergency room.

People allergic to	May react to
tree pollen	cherries, apricots, kiwis, oranges, plums, hazelnuts, and walnuts
grass pollen	melons, tomatoes, and oranges
oak or birch pollen	carrots, celery, almonds, apples, peaches, and pears
ragweed	bananas, cantaloupe, cucumber, zucchini, and chamomile tea

Buyer beware: 'hypoallergenic' may be all hype

The term "hypoallergenic" belongs entirely to the marketing world. The claim is not regulated by the Food and Drug Administration (FDA), which means companies can stick a hypoallergenic label on anything.

To find out how the claims stack up in run-of-the-mill goods, scientists put it to the test. They evaluated allergens in 187 products marketed as "hypoallergenic," "dermatologist recommended/tested," "fragrance free," or "paraben free." They found that 89 percent contained at least one allergen — the most common were preservatives and fragrances.

Outsmart food allergies with fiber

An Australian study reports a high-fiber diet, along with the right amount of vitamin A, could help protect against food allergies by actually changing the type and amount of bacteria in your gut. Children, especially, are prone to food allergies, and the researchers believe if their diet falls short of these important nutrients, they could be at risk. No matter what your age, a healthy amount of fiber is good for your digestion and your immune system. So make sure you get enough by loading your plate with plenty of fruits and vegetables.

Avoid herbs that add to your woes

Be careful about drinking herbal teas when you suffer from allergies. They may contain leaves or pollen you're sensitive to. For example, people take echinacea to help prevent colds, but it helps boost their immune system, not relieve symptoms. If your nose is stuffy and you think echinacea will help ease your congestion, you could be making a big mistake. It may actually worsen your symptoms or even trigger some you've never experienced before.

Going green is getting easier — and cheaper

Ever felt hot and itchy after slipping on freshly washed clothes? If so, you might have suffered an allergic reaction to the chemicals in your laundry detergent and opted for a more natural alternative.

Unfortunately, not every cleaner with an "earth-friendly" label is 100 percent safe for you and the environment. While lots of companies make claims that their products are natural and eco-friendly, not all deliver on their promises.

So how can you spot the real McCoy? Read labels and look for words like "solvent free" and "no phosphates."

Children from the former East Germany had more allergies when they were exposed to a Western lifestyle. Among the changes: more wall-to-wall carpet, damper homes, and more cats.

Spend the same greenbacks on green cleaners. Environmentally friendly and organic household cleaners now run in the same general price range — from about 7 to 19 cents an ounce — as competing products that contain chemicals and preservatives.

So with price no longer an issue, why else should you lean towards green?

▸ Health. Harsh chemicals can irritate the skin and trigger allergies and asthma. Cutting back on regular exposure lowers your chances of becoming ill.

▸ Home. Synthetic soap and detergents contain active agents — dubbed surfactants — that help lift off and wash away dirt. Modern surfactants are often petroleum-based or made with animal fat and contribute to the formation of soap film, or scum. Believe it or not, using too much detergent can cause gummy buildup, mold, or mildew in your appliances. That's why it's best to choose plant-based products whenever possible.

▸ Environment. The less toxic your waste water is, the more likely your local treatment center can properly clean it for reuse.

Do green products really clean as well? When one independent organization compared the cleaning power behind several all-purpose household sprays, both green and regular, their results were mixed. In some cases, green products held their own in basic cleaning tasks compared with more conventional cleaners.

But what if you're set on buying environmentally safe products? You can find the Environmental Protection Agency's Safer Choice product list at *epa.gov/saferchoice*. In addition, the Environmental Working Group provides a guide to healthy cleaning products at *ewg.org/guides/cleaners*. Both lists are updated regularly.

To make your consumer dollars count, read labels. Manufacturers are not required to list the chemicals in their cleaners, but they should tell you if their products are dangerous. Pay special attention to labels with product warnings and health hazards.

You want to use products that carry these kinds of labels:

▸ non-toxic

▸ biodegradable

▸ bleach-free

▸ dye-free

▸ petroleum-free

▸ chlorine-free

▸ made from renewable resources

▸ scented with natural plant derivatives or essential oils

Alzheimer's disease
Get treatment without breaking the bank

Alzheimer's disease (AD) is a type of dementia that slowly destroys memory and mental abilities. It affects over 5 million people just in the United States, but that number is estimated to nearly triple in the next 40 years. The heartbreak of AD is that while there is no cure, it is possible for a loved one to live for decades with the disease. The Alzheimer's Association estimates the total lifetime cost of caring for someone with AD is greater than $357,000.

Researchers are working hard to discover a better treatment for Alzheimer's disease, but in the meantime, know your options. The good news is some drugs can help manage AD or slow down the process. The better news is certain lifestyle changes can lower your risk of getting the disease in the first place.

Read on to learn what medications work, which ones you should avoid, and what can help you manage this condition.

Eat right to protect your memories

What you eat can affect every aspect of your health, and it turns out eating a Mediterranean diet rich in fruits, vegetables, and fish can reduce your risk of Alzheimer's disease.

Columbia University researchers surveyed over 2,000 people aged 65 and over and found the ones who ate foods from the Mediterranean diet were 40 percent less likely to develop Alzheimer's. Follow their lead with these helpful foods.

Try the catch of the day. Fish is the entrée of choice when it comes to healthy hearts and minds. It is low in harmful saturated fat and high in healthy unsaturated fats like omega-3 fatty acids. In one study of seniors, those that ate fish at least once a week were 60 percent less likely to develop Alzheimer's disease compared to those who rarely ate fish. Good sources of healthy omega-3 fatty acids include salmon, halibut, mackerel, and sardines, but you can also get it from walnuts, almonds, and soy.

Eat your fruits and vegetables. Energize your brain naturally without dangerous drugs. Jump-start it with the folate you get from foods like broccoli, spinach, asparagus, beans, papaya, and orange juice. Scientists studied 300 older men and found that eating folate-rich foods protected them from declines in memory and thinking skills.

Pour a glass of wine. It doesn't make sense to start drinking alcohol for your health, but wine in moderation can be good for you. Red wine, especially, has resveratrol — a chemical found in grapes that reduces the protein that causes damaging plaque in your brain. Red wine has more resveratrol than white wine, and Pinot Noir has the most of all.

Watch out for memory-stealing drugs

The medicine you're taking for high blood pressure, asthma, allergies, pain, nausea, irregular heartbeat, ulcers, or Parkinson's disease may be stealing your memory. Anticholinergic drugs are prescribed for conditions like these because they block a certain neurotransmitter — a chemical that regulates nerve impulses. While these drugs help control your heart, or your breathing, or your muscles, for example, they can also inhibit memory. So, if you feel your attention, recall, or reaction time is suffering, it may not be dementia at all.

Sidestep AD with common meds

While some drugs are accepted treatments for Alzheimer's symptoms, there are other options you might not have considered.

Lower your cholesterol and your Alzheimer's risk. The medicine you may already be taking could be the key to preventing Alzheimer's. Statins — drugs that keep your cholesterol levels down — could help you avoid this dreaded disease. Studies have shown that Alzheimer's patients who regularly took statins experienced a slower mental decline along with lower cholesterol.

Manage BP to slow dementia. Got high blood pressure? Don't wait to deal with it. Research shows that for every year you treat this damaging condition, your risk of dementia goes down three percent. If you're already taking a potassium-sparing diuretic there's more good news — you may be lowering your risk of Alzheimer's by up to 70 percent. This medicine helps your body hang on to potassium, a mineral that allows your brain to send signals between nerves. And no matter what, control your numbers — avoid large swings in blood pressure readings throughout the day. Japanese researchers think big changes can lead to more memory lapses.

Although not everyone agrees controlling blood pressure decreases your risk of dementia, it's such a smart move anyway that even a slight chance of Alzheimer's prevention is a nice bonus.

Black currants and boysenberries may protect your brain from Alzheimer's disease with potent compounds called anthocyanins and polyphenolics. British black currants have the most benefit because they're darker.

Take two aspirin and remember me in the morning. Most experts agree inflammation plays a role in the development of Alzheimer's. That's why, in theory, preventing AD with nonsteroidal anti-inflammatory drugs (NSAIDs) like aspirin, acetaminophen, or ibuprofen just makes sense. And even though not all clinical trials have proven this to be true, enough studies on long-term use are positive to keep the research community interested. Talk to your doctor about NSAIDs because there are potential side effects.

Save that thought with helpful herbs

Drugs aren't the only way to improve your memory. Natural herbs and supplements can help, too.

Put the kettle on. It tastes good, it's inexpensive, and you know it's healthy. Now, it could save your memory, too. It's green tea, and it contains an antioxidant called epigallocatechin-3-gallate. Otherwise known as EGCG, this natural ingredient kept harmful, sticky plaques from forming on the brains of mice that had been engineered to develop AD. Drink three to four cups a day of decaffeinated green tea for the most benefit. Steep a teaspoon of leaves or a tea bag in one cup of boiling water for three minutes. Then strain and enjoy.

Aged garlic attacks AD-causing compounds. Whenever you get a cut or scrape, your body heals itself. And your brain is no different. If it's hurt by pollutants, trauma, or age-related stress, it activates microglial cells, your natural form of damage control. These cells gather and multiply to stop injuries from getting worse and to kick-start the healing process.

But there's a problem. Microglial cells also produce nitric oxide (NO), a chemical compound which, in excess, experts think leads to AD.

Researchers from the University of Missouri believe one secret to preventing this dangerous domino effect is in garlic—specifically aged garlic. A compound created during the aging process, called fructosyl arginine (FruArg), actually stops the production of NO. If you can't find aged garlic extract as a supplement at your local store, it's available for sale online.

A natural way to get this compound is from an exotic ingredient called black garlic. This sweet, mellow spice is just regular garlic that's been aged until the cloves turn black. Track it down at local grocers or buy black garlic on the internet.

Let Medicare foot the bill

Early detection of Alzheimer's is critical to starting a drug treatment program that will help hold off the disease. Unfortunately, it's very hard to identify in its initial stages. Enter the PET — positron emission tomography — scan. This powerful brain scan correctly diagnoses Alzheimer's about 90 percent of the time. The problem is one scan often costs around $5,000. But if you know someone whose dementia has been getting worse for six months, Medicare may cover the cost. Check it out because private health insurance companies may already be following suit.

Ping-pong isn't just a way to kill time. In one study, playing the game increased blood flow to the brain and decreased symptoms in dementia patients — regardless of how well they played.

Support eases caregiving burden

No man is an island. Taking care of someone with Alzheimer's disease is a big job and can become overwhelming if you take it on by yourself.

A recent study shows that when family caregivers work as a team to look after an Alzheimer's patient, it not only helps the caregiver feel less stressed, but also improves dementia symptoms

India may have the world's lowest rate of Alzheimer's because of curry. Curcumin, the spice's yellow pigment, keeps beta-amyloid plaques from forming and even breaks down existing plaques.

in the patient. Another study found that symptoms were also better in patients whose caregivers felt less depressed and burdened. It's OK to ask for help and support. You're doing the patient a favor by taking care of yourself as much as you take care of them.

If you need a break to recharge, take advantage of a respite program — a service provided by organizations to help people who provide care to chronically ill senior citizens. Sometimes they'll give you free care services or grants, or they'll at least put you in contact with services you fund yourself. Use the Eldercare Locator to find a respite program near you. Go online at *https://eldercare.acl.gov* or call 800-677-1116.

Geriatric care managers are another option. They help people make sense of nursing homes, insurance policies, legal issues, medications, and other confusing aspects of home care.

Simple test an early clue to Alzheimer's

People in the early stages of Alzheimer's disease have trouble recalling certain words. In a study at the University of York in Great Britain, participants were asked to name as many animals as they could in one minute. Researchers discovered that the Alzheimer's victims remembered words learned early in life, like dog and cat, but had difficulty recalling words learned later, like leopard.

This simple test could help determine if someone is suffering from a memory lapse or Alzheimer's disease.

Better, smarter, faster: The real secret to staying young

Would you believe something as simple as searching for items in an unfamiliar store can sharpen your memory and problem-solving skills? The act of walking and thinking at the same time benefits you more than mental exercise alone.

Aerobic exercise floods your brain cells with oxygen and nutrients. That may be why physical activity can speed your thinking and help you process information faster. It also helps keep your blood vessels from hardening, including those in your brain. Experts think that may be a key reason some people stay mentally sharp as they age.

Working on puzzles and games is a great way to stay mentally fit. But the real secret to boosting your brain is working out the rest of your body, too.

Although most people's brains shrink somewhat as they age, those who have a genetic marker for Alzheimer's disease tend to lose even more volume in the hippocampus, the region of the brain dealing with memory and learning. But moderate exercise seems to have a protective effect.

"We found that physical activity has the potential to preserve the volume of the hippocampus in those with increased risk for Alzheimer's disease," says Dr. J. Carson Smith, a researcher at the University of Maryland School of Public Health. "That means we can possibly delay cognitive decline and the onset of dementia symptoms in these individuals."

Healthy teeth and gums may mean more than a nice smile. Researchers have found that inflammation and infection caused by loose teeth can quadruple your risk of Alzheimer's disease.

Other studies also tout the protective effects of exercise. Dutch scientists found that regular aerobic exercise boosted the size of the hippocampus in women with mild memory problems. And research out of Finland showed that people who exercised twice a week had a lower risk of dementia than those who were less active, even if they started after middle age.

Awaken to a better life — how this natural remedy protects your brain

Did you know that sleep plays an important role in the consolidation of memories? It's essential for learning new things. So if you don't sleep well or can't doze off, you could be setting yourself up for a decline in cognitive performance.

Insomnia is a common problem among older folks, in part because the production of melatonin — a hormone that regulates the sleep-wake cycle — declines with age. But here's the good news. Melatonin supplements may be able to restore your sleep cycle — and the sleep cycles of people with dementia — to normal. That's what scientists found when they tested the effects of the hormone on seniors who were taking medication to treat mild to moderate AD.

Eighty participants took either 2 milligrams (mg) of melatonin or a placebo one to two hours before bedtime for 24 weeks. By the end of the study, the melatonin group was able to sleep for longer lengths of time than the placebo group. They also performed better on tests measuring their cognitive function.

Dollars&Sense
9 smart ways to slash health-care costs

Health-care costs have been rising five times faster than salaries. Use these tips to help shrink your spending and get more bang for your medical buck.

Save at in-store clinics. These walk-in clinics are opening up at Walmarts, drugstores, and other retailers. They're much cheaper than doctors' offices — some say half as much — and significantly less than the emergency room. Many of these clinics only treat minor illnesses, but their nurse practitioners can refer you to a doctor if you need further care.

Get health-care assistance. If you have no insurance or can't pay for health care, visit *hrsa.gov* or call toll-free 877-464-4772. You'll learn about centers that offer low- or no-cost emergency exams, lab tests, X-rays, and immunizations. This program does not cover medication costs.

Choose insurance wisely. Don't pick an insurance plan solely because the premiums are low. Co-payments and deductibles can cost you a lot. So can choosing a plan that doesn't match your needs. For example, a PPO-style plan is often more economical for people who expect to use specialists or out-of-network doctors. But if your family rarely gets sick and only needs check-ups and preventive care, an HMO-style plan may be best.

Pay with tax-free dollars. Stash them in a flexible spending account (FSA.) New rules give you 10 extra weeks after December 31 to use up each year's contributions to your account, so you're less likely to forfeit leftover money at deadline time. And now you can spend FSA dollars on nonprescription drugs, insurance deductibles and co-payments, flu shots, and more. Ask your plan administrator which expenses qualify.

Avoid preventable costs. Specialists like allergists or gastroenterologists can be expensive on some insurance plans. Before you visit a specialist, call and check with your family doctor first. She can help you determine whether the extra cost of a specialist is necessary.

Screen your medical tests. The U.S. Preventive Services Task Force says some screenings and tests should not be given to healthy people unless a doctor has reason to suspect disease. These tests are less likely to uncover hidden disease in symptom-free people and more likely to produce inaccurate results that require more testing. But new research shows that doctors still order these tests. Before agreeing to a test, ask why you need it and how it will affect treatment decisions. You may discover the test isn't necessary.

Choose outpatient surgery. You could save hundreds by avoiding an overnight hospital stay. Ask your doctor about the risks and benefits of outpatient surgery.

Catch billing errors. Most medical bills contain at least one error. While you're in the hospital, ask family members to help you keep a log of all tests, medication, and procedures that you're given. Then request an itemized bill from the hospital. Compare it with your log, and check for double billings, items you didn't get, or inaccurate dates. If you find a problem, notify both your insurance company and a hospital billing department supervisor.

Volunteer for a clinical trial. You can try new medicines and treatments that may not be available otherwise. The treatment under study is generally free, but ask to make sure. You can find industry-funded clinical trials in your area online at *www.centerwatch.com*. To learn about government-sponsored clinical trials, visit *www.clinicaltrials.gov*, or ask for help at your doctor's office or local clinic. Visit *www.cc.nih.gov* or call the Patient Recruitment Office at 800-411-1222 for studies at the National Institutes of Health Clinical Center in Bethesda, Maryland.

Anxiety

Low-cost ways to calm jangled nerves

Everyone worries occasionally. Your family, health, and financial situation — to name just a few aspects of everyday life — can cause plenty of legitimate concerns. But some people worry almost all the time. For people with generalized anxiety disorder (GAD), the most common form of anxiety, life can be overwhelming.

Excessive worrying, tension, and feelings of dread accompany your day-to-day decisions. You probably realize your worrying is way out of proportion to the situation, but you can't help agonizing over it. This constant feeling of being on edge takes its toll on your quality of life. In fact, anxiety often leads to physical symptoms, like headaches, sweating, palpitations, nausea, restlessness, and sleep disturbances.

When you are anxious, you have enough worries. One thing you shouldn't have to worry about is finding ways to feel better. Try these simple strategies to battle stress and reduce anxiety levels.

Seek expert help to get back on track

Drugs certainly have their place in treating anxiety. The right prescription can help you function and feel like yourself again.

But maybe you don't need drugs at all. Instead of relying on a "magic pill" to make you feel better, try getting to the root of your problems with therapy.

Cognitive behavioral therapy, with its focus on helping you change how you think about and react to stressful situations, is considered the best option for generalized anxiety disorder. Look for a qualified therapist. You may want to ask your doctor for a recommendation.

Remember, drugs and therapy are not mutually exclusive. You don't have to choose one or the other. In fact, combining your medication with therapy can make your treatment even more effective.

What time is it? Time to ease your tension. Stressed-out British politicians found that wearing a magnetic wrist-watch helped relieve anxiety and improve their sleep.

Just talking about your problems with other people, perhaps in a support group, can also help. Thanks to the Internet, you can even chat with a therapist online.

Melt your cares away with a massage

Take a hands-on approach to relieving your anxiety — get a massage. There's nothing like a good rubdown to eliminate tension and stress.

Swedish massage is the most common type, and a typical massage can cost $50 to $130 an hour. Sometimes your insurance will even cover the cost if it's for medical reasons.

Massage is an effective alternative treatment. Just make sure you find a qualified massage therapist. You can do that at the American Massage Therapy Association Web site at *www.amtamassage.org*.

Hands-on therapies, like massage, might not be best for everyone, including people who suffer from panic attacks.

Another good way to relieve mild anxiety is through aromatherapy. Often used in conjunction with massage, aromatherapy involves soothing scents from essential oils. Some favorites include lavender, chamomile, and jasmine.

Straight talk about natural alternatives

Herbs and supplements provide natural alternatives to prescription medication. But natural does not always mean safe.

For example, the herb kava does help relieve anxiety. But it also comes with some risks, including the possibility of liver damage. So while it might be effective, it may not be the best option.

Other herbs that have been used to treat anxiety include passion flower and gotu kola, but more research needs to be done before they can be recommended. For mild stress relief, you can also turn to valerian, ginseng, or chamomile. Supplements that may help your body deal with stress include vitamin C, B vitamins, and magnesium.

Holding hands helps lower anxiety. In a recent study, brain scans of women anticipating an electric shock showed a soothing effect when their husbands held their hands.

Unlike prescription drugs, the Food and Drug Administration (FDA) does not regulate herbs and supplements. That means you do not always know exactly what you're getting. Always tell your doctor what herbs you're taking. Certain herbs may dangerously interact with drugs.

Smart way to calm an anxious mind

What you put on your plate may affect what goes on in your mind. That's why a healthy diet may play a role in overcoming anxiety.

In times of stress, your body especially needs protein. Complex carbohydrates, vitamin C, B vitamins, and minerals like zinc, iron, and selenium will also serve you well.

One study found that eating gazpacho, a cold vegetable soup, helped lower stress chemicals in the body. Other specific foods that may help reduce stress include asparagus, broccoli, kale, and spinach, which are chock-full of B vitamins. Warm milk may also calm your nerves.

Omega-3 fatty acids, found in fish, walnuts, and flaxseed, can have a calming effect, especially if you also cut down on omega-6 fatty acids, which appear in vegetable oils and deep-fried or processed foods.

Explore the world of unusual phobias

Phobia, the excessive and persistent fear of a specific object or situation, is a common anxiety disorder. You've probably heard of agoraphobia, the fear of open spaces, or xenophobia, the fear of foreigners or strangers. But what about arachibutyrophobia? That's the fear of peanut butter sticking to the roof of your mouth. Pogonophobia is the fear of beards, while syngenesophobia is the fear of relatives. For more interesting phobias, check out the Phobia List at *www.phobialist.com*.

Avoid caffeine and alcohol, which can adversely affect your mood and leave you jittery or depressed. They can also lessen the effects of some anxiety medications.

Breathe in some peace of mind

Take a deep breath, count to 10, and feel your worries fall away. Well, that's how it's supposed to work. In reality, you may have to practice more control over your breathing, and do it for longer than a count of 10. But the basic idea holds — you can change the way you breathe to get control of your stress level.

Deep breathing helps you relax. You take about 14 to 16 breaths each minute while you are at rest. But when you are in a stressful situation, you tend to breathe faster as your lungs work to take in more oxygen as part of the fight-or-flight response.

Here's how deep breathing helps. When you breathe deeply, you work your diaphragm, the powerful sheet of muscle that separates your lungs from your stomach. Taking a deep breath lowers your diaphragm, pulling your lungs down with it and pressing against organs in your abdomen to make room for your lungs to expand as they fill with air. Then as you breathe out, your diaphragm presses up against your lungs, pushing out carbon dioxide. This kind of deep breathing engages what is called the "relaxation response." That is the opposite of the stress response.

Research shows that practicing deep-breathing exercises can lower your anxiety, stress, and depression while it increases your feelings of optimism. It's free and safe stress relief, and you can do it anywhere, at any time.

Follow the path to stress relief. Find time to do these deep-breathing exercises several times each day, even if you don't feel especially stressed. First, inhale through your nose slowly and deeply, counting to 10. Be sure your stomach and abdomen expand, but your chest does not. Then, exhale through your nose slowly, also while you count to 10. Concentrate on counting and breathing through each cycle to quiet your mind. Repeat the cycle five to 10 times.

Boost your mood with a little creativity

Adult coloring books are the new craze in America. Fans of this hobby claim it relieves stress and helps them relax. But is there any science behind getting crafty to fight anxiety?

While most evidence comes from personal testimonies, a few small studies do show that crafts such as knitting help calm anxiety. Many find that the repetitive motion and focus required for these tasks are quite soothing.

Doing crafts can take your mind off worries, quiet your nerves, and give you a sense of pride. So make time for what makes you happy, whether it's knitting, painting, or scrapbooking.

Take a bite out of stress with a tasty chew

Oh, the delicious chewing gums of youth. Remember Fruit Stripe? Doublemint? How about Wrigley's Spearmint? You slipped a stick into your mouth before every math test, hoping the eagle-eyed teacher wouldn't see. You didn't know it then, but chewing on that tasty wad probably helped your algebra anxiety go way down. So will a couple of Chiclets still work to lower your stress today?

It seems almost unbelievable, but you can actually reduce fatigue, anxiety, and depression with a good chew. That's according to a study of more than 100 volunteers carried out at Cardiff University in Wales. And Japanese researchers from a separate study add one additional note — they discovered the harder you chew, the greater your stress relief. That study also said participants only had to chew for three minutes before their stress hormones went down.

So why does chewing gum work this way? Some parts of the brain like the hippocampus — the region in the brain that regulates your emotions and responds to stress — function differently when you're chewing. In fact, researchers think just the simple act of chewing may get the messenger cells in your hippocampus riled up enough to tamp down your stress and anxiety.

No need to look for a special gum. Any of your favorites will do the trick. Just sit back, relax, and chew away your stress.

Simple steps to squash stress

They may not be as powerful as prescription drugs or therapy, but these simple lifestyle strategies can help reduce your stress.

- **Get plenty of sleep each night.** Your body needs to recharge.
- **Laugh more.** Watch a funny movie or visit a humorous friend or relative. Studies show laughter lowers stress.
- **Exercise regularly.** You'll sleep better, feel better about yourself, and reduce anxiety symptoms.
- **Spend time in your garden.** It's a peaceful way to get some exercise.
- **Play some music.** Whether you tickle the ivories on your piano or just turn on the radio, music helps you relax.
- **Hold no grudges.** Forgiveness helps lower stress — and the health problems that come with it.
- **Take a vacation.** It may seem obvious, but just getting away for a vacation will do wonders for your health.

▸ **Affirm your values.** A recent study of college students found that those who reflected on values important to them, such as religion or social issues, before undertaking a stressful task had lower levels of the stress hormone cortisol.

Let nature relax, refresh, and restore

Ready for a stroll? Head for the park, not downtown. Take the green path, not the sidewalk.

Maybe soaking up the atmosphere of nature, which the Japanese call forest bathing, has always made you feel better, but now science proves it can lessen anxiety and negative thinking. A peaceful stroll through the woods may also lower symptoms of stress by balancing your heart rate, blood pressure, and stress hormones.

A walk in the woods can also be a spiritual experience. So take that time to engage in some private prayer and it may restore your health if you're struggling with depression or anxiety.

Asthma

How to control symptoms — and cost

About 25 million Americans have asthma, and thousands — many of them elderly — die from it every year. About 15 percent of all people who have asthma are over 65, when asthma attacks can combine with other health problems to make things worse.

Asthma is a chronic inflammation of your airways that tightens up your bronchial tubes and fills them with mucus. Unfortunately, it has some of the same symptoms as several other diseases, including heart attack. You need a doctor's diagnosis to be sure of what you have.

Once you know you have asthma, get the most for the money you spend on treatment by working closely with your doctor to get the right dosage of the right medicine. You'll find asthma-fighting tips throughout this chapter.

Top foods that fight asthma

Studies show that people who eat a lot of the right kind of foods are less likely to have asthma. Vegetables, fruit, and fish are all part of a good defense against breathing problems.

Go to the garden for vitamins. Carrots, tomatoes, and leafy greens like lettuce and spinach are rich in carotenoids. These phytonutrients convert to vitamin A, which helps regulate your immune system and keep the lining of your respiratory tract in shape.

Sweet peppers, especially the red ones, are another good asthma-fighting vegetable. They have lots of vitamin C, the major antioxidant in the surface of the lungs. Just one cup of red peppers will give you 283 milligrams of vitamin C — more than three times your daily requirement. Oranges and other citrus fruits are also good choices for this important nutrient.

Eat apples to avoid asthma. They're red and delicious, and they top the list of fruits that may ease asthma. Apples are full of quercetin and other flavonoid antioxidants that fight the free radicals produced by your inflamed airways. Apple peelings have even more quercetin than the flesh, so be sure and eat all the apple.

Build up your lungs with fish. Researchers think the omega-3 fatty acids in fish oil may help your lungs by suppressing inflammation. Studies have shown that eating fish seems to help more than taking fish oil supplements. Experts recommend eating fish three or more times a week as part of a well-balanced diet that keeps up your levels of omega-3.

The little pill you should never take

You may reach for aspirin when you're in pain, but research shows that may not be a good idea if you're asthmatic. Over-the-counter (OTC) pain relievers will set off an attack in about one of every five adult asthma sufferers.

Experts call it aspirin-induced asthma, but it includes other nonsteroidal anti-inflammatory drugs (NSAIDs) like ibuprofen and naproxen as well. If you think this has happened to you, you should switch to the non-NSAID painkiller acetaminophen, some experts say. Unfortunately, research also links the regular use of acetaminophen with increased asthma risk, so it's possible that could cause problems as well.

Cold remedies and even heartburn medicines often contain pain relievers, too. Read the labels of all over-the-counter medicines and know exactly what you are taking. Don't forget to tell your doctor about all the medicines, herbs, and supplements you take whenever you get a new prescription.

Remember, too, that pills aren't the only answers for aches and pains. You can avoid both the side effects and expense of painkilling drugs by first trying ice packs, heating pads, physical activity, or relaxation.

Help yourself during an attack

Pursed-lip breathing can help keep your airways open during an asthma attack. Breathe in through your nose and out through your mouth with your lips in a whistling or kissing position. Take two seconds to inhale and four to six seconds to exhale.

5 ways to guard against EIA

Don't be afraid to exercise if you have asthma. Working out can boost your breathing capacity and cut back on asthma symptoms. Even the American Thoracic Society recommends moderate aerobic exercise for asthmatics. But don't go overboard. Before you start training, take steps to guard against the possibility of exercise-induced asthma (EIA).

Vigorous physical activity triggers asthma attacks in more than 90 percent of people who have asthma. About 10 percent of the general population, some of whom don't normally have asthma, also suffer attacks. EIA may be even more common among serious athletes. Studies of Olympians have shown up to 40 percent suffer EIA symptoms.

These steps will help you avoid this potentially serious problem.

▸ Make sure you have your overall asthma under control.

▸ Take a dose of your albuterol inhaler 15 to 30 minutes before you work out.

▸ Exercise in a warm, humid environment.

▸ Include warm-up and cool-down periods in your workout.

▸ Avoid salt in your diet, and eat plenty of foods with antioxidants and omega-3 fatty acids. Caffeine also helps reduce the severity of EIA.

Stop bringing home the bacon and breathe easier

Country-fried ham, bacon, and sausage might sound like the start of an amazing Saturday morning breakfast, but they could also be an invitation to an asthma attack.

Researchers found in a study of over 35,000 people that eating processed meat was associated with more asthma symptoms, especially when participants were overweight, eating a lower quality diet, or smoking.

Why? For one, when you eat cured meats, the amount of C-reactive proteins in your body goes up, which means more inflammation and possibly more trouble breathing. To make things worse, cured meats are packed with three ingredients that aggravate asthma.

▸ **Nitrites.** These are preservatives that prolong the shelf life of your meat. While nitrites alone are not the bad guys, they can turn on you in a flash when cooked in high heat. That's when they convert to nitrosamines, which may cause inflammation in your airways.

▸ **Advanced glycation end products (AGEs).** These blood vessel-clogging compounds are found naturally in animal products and increase when the meat is cooked and processed. As they build up in your system, they contribute to lung inflammation. One study says that may be why eating meat is linked to breathing problems. Use an acidic marinade with a lemon or vinegar base on your meat to keep AGEs from forming when you cook.

▸ **Salt.** Since the '30s, studies have shown that high-salt diets increase asthma symptoms, but lowering the salt seems to decrease them.

How much is too much? A French study of nearly 1,000 participants over an average of seven years offers some insight. Those who ate more than three servings per week of cured meat like ham and sausage experienced worsening asthma symptoms over time. But for overall health benefits, experts at Harvard recommend limiting processed meats to once or twice a month.

Avoid lung-damaging aroma

Stop buying mothballs, air fresheners, and toilet bowl deodorizers. You'll not only save money, you may save your lungs. Scientists have found that the chemical you smell in mothballs affects lung function, which can be serious if you have asthma. The volatile organic compound 1,4-dichlorobenzene (1,4-DCB) is a prime ingredient in many sanitizing products. Control the risk from 1,4-DCB by limiting your use of these items.

No matter how you slice it, eating less processed meat may help reduce your asthma symptoms, but experts still caution you not to stop using your inhaler.

Natural solutions keep asthma at bay

You can help yourself avoid asthma attacks naturally. Try boosting your breathing with these nutrients and herbs.

Magnesium is a natural bronchodilator. It helps open up your airways and ease the muscle spasms of asthma attacks. You can keep up the magnesium level in your body by eating avocados, oysters, beans, and broccoli.

> Laughter is a more common asthma trigger than even dust mites and mold. Experts think it may have to do with hyperventilation.

Rosemary is an herb used for flavoring food and beverages, but it has also been used in folk medicine as an antispasmodic. It relaxes the smooth muscles of the trachea and reduces the production of leukotrienes that cause inflammation. Research shows that a mixture of Chinese herbs called anti-asthma herbal medicine intervention (ASHMI) may be as safe and effective in treating moderate asthma as the corticosteroid prednisone — without the side effects.

Butterbur extract helps control asthma and hay fever by acting as an antihistamine and improving lung function. Certain parts of this plant can be harmful, but the extracts used in research had no toxins. Be careful though. Butterbur is primarily a European medicine that is not regulated in the United States, so some products on the market may not be safe to use. It's best to talk to your doctor about any herbal remedies you would like to try.

Avoid dried fruits to win the war against asthma

Fruit is good for you, right? Well, yes. But if you have asthma, you may be sensitive to a sneaky ingredient that can be found in dried fruit — sulfites.

Sulfites are sulfur-based compounds that are added to foods to boost flavors and preserve freshness. In addition to dried fruit, they can be found in wine, white grape juice, shrimp, maraschino cherries, jams and jellies, and many other products.

Sulfites can cause allergic reactions, especially if you have asthma. About three to 10 percent of people with asthma have a sulfite sensitivity. If you experience chest tightness, stomach cramps, diarrhea, hives, or breathing problems when you eat foods containing sulfite, you too may be sensitive to the additive.

Breathe easy with this 'E'ssential vitamin

You take over 670 million breaths by the time you reach the age of 80. But what if you have asthma or some other lung condition? Every breath you take is a struggle. It doesn't have to be. Thanks to vitamin E, your lungs can get a second wind.

Vitamin E is a fat-soluble nutrient made up of eight related substances. Experts say two of these — alpha-tocopherol and gamma-tocopherol — can affect your breathing.

Eat corn, soybean, or canola oil and you're getting gamma-tocopherol. This form of

Asthmatics may soon benefit from their own "music therapy." Researchers are studying how playing wind instruments like flutes and horns can increase lung capacity.

vitamin E makes your lungs work harder, suggests a Northwestern University study. Scientists say when gamma-tocopherol binds with a special protein called kinase C-alpha, it increases inflammation in your lungs.

But when this protein binds with alpha-tocopherol, inflammation clears up. You can find alpha-tocopherol in oils like olive, almond, sunflower, and wheat germ, plus nuts, seeds, and leafy green vegetables.

Researchers also noted that countries with low rates of asthma eat a lot more olive and sunflower oils than in America. The rate of asthma in the U.S. has climbed over the past 40 years, and coincides with higher use of corn, soybean, and canola oils.

Protect health with an ozone-free home

An air purifier in your home might be just the ticket if airborne allergens are a major factor in triggering your asthma. They can filter out triggers like pollen, mold, dust, and animal dander. But avoid air cleaners that produce ozone — either on purpose or incidentally. While ozone is great for purifying water or blocking ultraviolet rays, it is also the primary ingredient of smog and can make your asthma much worse. See the *Allergies* chapter to learn more about choosing the best type of air cleaner for your condition.

Back pain

Right techniques promise real relief

There are two kinds of people — those with back problems and those without. In the United States alone, back injuries cost more than $80 billion a year in medical expenses and lost work.

Roughly four out of five people will suffer with back pain at some point during their lives. Too often, doctors don't know why. In an effort to end your pain, they may prescribe surgery you don't need or pain medications that cause serious health problems.

But here is something you may not know — in nine out of 10 cases, back injuries heal on their own within six weeks. Ahead, you'll discover easy-does-it secrets to help you escape back pain and — surprise — none of them calls for surgery, drugs, or extra time in bed.

Try some free (and fun) therapy

Physical therapy can help you get on your feet after a lingering back injury, but emerging evidence suggests you can save money and get the same pain-busting benefits with do-it-yourself workouts.

Ask for advice. Your doctor may refer you for physical therapy if your pain lasts longer than three weeks. Instead of signing up for weeks of costly therapy, ask about a one-time session for exercise advice. In a study published in the prestigious *British Medical Journal,* advice from a physical therapist on how to stay active helped people with mild to moderate low back pain as much as four or more weeks of physical therapy.

Make fitness fun. Leisurely, low-impact workouts like walking and swimming seem to relieve low back pain better than specific back exercises. Fun activities like these also lighten psychological stress. In fact, researchers from the University of California and University of Michigan say walking briskly about half an hour each day is enough to reap these pain-reducing, mood-boosting benefits. Doing specific back exercises, on the other hand, may worsen both back pain and stress.

Turn up the heat. Applying heat with a Thermacare patch, heating pad, or hot, moist compress can cut pain even more. Exercising and wearing a continuous low-level heat wrap for five days packed more pain relief and improved function better than exercise or heat wraps alone in a study of 100 people with acute low back pain. What's more, 72 percent of those who used this combo treatment regained full mobility just one week after starting it.

After a back injury, you should try to return to your normal activities as soon as possible, as much as your pain allows. Simply start out slow to give damaged muscles time to rebuild.

Surgery: a last resort for bad backs

Few people truly need back surgery. In fact, some experts say less than 1 percent of people with back pain need aggressive surgery. In most cases, natural alternatives like exercise, physical therapy, and applying heat and cold help heal the injury. If your doctor tells you that you need surgery, get a second opinion.

If you suffer with sciatic pain, worsening weakness in the legs, or a herniated disc or spinal stenosis (narrowing of the spine) causing bowel or bladder control problems, you may need surgery if medicines and natural options don't help after six weeks. Discuss your particular case with a doctor you trust, and choose a surgeon who has lots of experience performing the procedure you need. Remember, surgery is not always successful, it may take months to fully heal, and you may never regain full flexibility.

Your back is particularly vulnerable when you first get out of bed. Go easy on it. Roll onto your side, bend your knees, push yourself upright with your arms, and lower your legs over the bedside.

End pain through proper posture

Here is a free, easy way to relieve back pain — improve your posture. Bad posture can worsen existing pain, but how you stand, sit, and even sleep could put the skip in your step again.

Stand tall. When standing, raise your head so your chin is parallel to the floor, and use your abdominal muscles to pull in your stomach. Don't stand "at attention," with shoulders pulled back and chin thrust out. This position only adds to back strain. Instead, keep your ears, shoulders, hips, knees, and ankles in line with each other. Try not to stand for long periods of time. If you do, take turns resting each foot on a nearby footstool.

Sit pretty. Sitting puts the most strain on your back, so get up and move every half hour. Choose straight-backed chairs or those with low-back support, and sit with your shoulders touching the chair back. Keep your upper back straight and chest lifted. If you spend lots of time at a desk, get a swivel chair that lets you turn without twisting at the waist. Look, too, for one with armrests and an adjustable back. You can place a rolled-up towel in the small of your back for added lumbar support. Sit with your knees slightly higher than your hips, and prop them on a footrest if needed.

Sleep smarter. Strategically placed pillows help support your back while you sleep. People with back pain should sleep on their side in a fetal position with a pillow between their knees to maintain the spine's natural curve. Back-sleepers, on the other hand, should put a pillow under their knees to support their lower back. Sleeping on your stomach is the worst position for a bad back and can trigger pain and prolong recovery. If you just can't break the habit, at least place a pillow under your stomach or chest to keep your spine aligned.

> To protect your stomach, look for buffered over-the-counter medications, and take them with food or milk.

Sleep your way to a better back

Doctors have long told people with bad backs to sleep on a hard mattress — but no more. Spanish researchers replaced the mattresses of 313 people with chronic low back pain with either soft, hard, or medium mattresses. Those who slept on the medium mattress for 90 days felt less pain and needed less pain medicine than those sleeping on a hard mattress.

That still leaves you lots of choices when bed shopping. Try this advice to narrow the field.

▶ **Don't trust tags.** They won't tell you how firm a mattress really is. One manufacturer's "firm" may be softer or harder than another's. Test each bed yourself by lying on it.

▶ **Buy the right size.** Single sleepers can make do with a twin bed, but couples need at least a queen-size so both people can move freely at night.

- **Don't go by price alone.** Buy the best quality mattress you can afford for longer-lasting sleep comfort.

- **Extend the life of your mattress.** Slip a piece of plywood between a too-soft mattress and its box spring. That will hold you over until you're ready to buy a new one.

Get crackin' to beat back problems

Chiropractic therapy, otherwise known as spinal manipulation, may help back pain that has lasted less than a month. Previous studies on its effectiveness have shown mixed results — it seems to help some people but not others. Now researchers think they have the answer why.

Army and Air Force physical therapists randomly assigned people with low back pain to either exercise therapy or spinal manipulation. Researchers also kept track of who improved with chiropractic treatment. People who met four out of five of these criteria were most likely to benefit.

- pain for fewer than 16 days
- only pain above the knees, not below
- not afraid of physical activity causing pain
- at least one stiff segment of the spine
- normal range of motion in at least one hip

Researchers say as many as 92 percent of people who meet four of the five criteria could improve after just one week of chiropractic treatment. Plus, six months later, people in the exercise-only group were taking more medicine, seeking more medical help, and had lost more work days due to back pain than those in the chiropractic group.

The sooner you seek help, the better. These experts say the single most accurate prediction of who would benefit from manipulation was how long their back pain had lasted.

A good doctor or chiropractor will first take X-rays and examine you for osteoporosis, herniated discs, spinal stenosis, and other nerve, bone, or joint disorders. People with these conditions are not candidates for chiropractic therapy.

Shockingly simple way to ease pain

Gentle jolts of electricity can help relieve pain. At least, that's the theory behind TENS (transcutaneous electric nerve stimulation) devices.

Visit a physical therapy clinic, and chances are you'll find one of these machines. TENS units have small electrodes that attach to your skin at or near the site of pain. The unit sends gentle electrical impulses that seem to block pain signals traveling to your brain, at least temporarily. It may also trigger your body to release natural feel-good chemicals called endorphins.

Short-term back pain is called acute. Pain that lasts longer than three months is considered chronic.

You can get TENS treatments in physical therapy or chiropractic offices, but buying or renting your own machine could save you a bundle, especially if you suffer with chronic back pain. In most cases, Medicare or insurance will help cover the cost.

Discuss TENS treatment with your doctor, and consider renting one first to see if it helps. Some devices are available for over-the-counter sale, but you will need a prescription to get Medicare or insurance coverage. Your doctor or physical therapist will also need to show you where to place the electrodes, how to operate the machine, and what settings to use for your pain.

Not all experts recommend TENS therapy, and it alone may not be enough to control back pain. It tends to work best in combination with other therapies, like pain relievers.

2 tried-and-true remedies tackle aches and pains

You're no stranger to pain. From the twinge of a pulled muscle to the constant ache of a sore back, you've spent more than your fair share of time suffering. A nice massage with soothing essential oils could be your remedy of choice. But if you need more easy solutions you can do yourself, try one of these other ways to send pain packing.

Explore aquatics. Water helps support your weight, putting less strain on your joints while offering gentle resistance. This makes water workouts, also called hydrotherapy, great for people with bone loss, joint pain, and muscle strains. Again, ask your doctor what activities are safe for your type of back pain.

Plank it out. A weak core puts your back in the injury danger zone. Do this exercise every day to strengthen your abdominal muscles and protect your back.

Important note — while the plank can minimize low back pain for many people, if you've suffered an injury, talk to your doctor or physical therapist before trying it.

▸ Get down on the floor, on your toes in the push-up position, with your hands shoulder-width apart.

▸ Keep your arms straight and your body in one long line.

▸ Contract all your muscles and hold for about 20 to 30 seconds.

▸ Rest and repeat.

If your back pain comes from scoliosis, a sideways curving of the spine, this classic side plank can help.

▸ Lie on your left side with your legs extended.

▸ Push up and straighten your left arm so you are supported by your left hand.

▸ Extend your right arm straight up, using a wall for support if needed.

▸ Raise your hips so your body is in a straight line from shoulders to ankles.

▸ Contract your stomach and leg muscles.

▸ Hold the position as long as possible, working up to 90 seconds.

▸ Repeat on your right side.

Is this classic side plank too difficult? Try a modified version where you rest on one elbow and keep your legs and hips on the floor, lifting only your upper body. Planking is easier than sit-ups, and as a bonus, it can help you flatten a bulging belly.

Get your back on track with yog-ahhh

Did you know that many people do exactly the wrong thing for back pain? They lay in bed, thinking rest is the best treatment.

The surprising truth is you should remain active to prevent muscle spasms and weakness in your back.

Although you want to avoid activities that worsen your pain, it's best to stay mobile and stick to your daily schedule as much as possible. If you must lie down, do so for only a few hours at a time.

Looking for quick relief? You'll be happy to hear yoga is just what the doctor ordered. That's according to scientists who evaluated 228 adults with chronic back pain. They divided participants into three groups, two of which participated in either yoga or intensive stretching in class and at home. The third group received a self-help book on pain management.

▸ At the end of three months, those in the yoga and stretching classes reported better back movement and less back pain than those in the self-help group. In fact, the two forms of exercise were equally effective.

▸ And, it turns out, the yoga and stretching groups had an easier time tossing out their pain pills. Compared with the self-care group, twice as many participants in the yoga and stretching classes reported lowering their medication use. That's great news for seniors, who need to be extra cautious about the potential side effects of opioid painkillers.

Beware of addictive drugs

Narcotic pain relievers such as OxyContin and Vicodin can work wonders for pain but can be addictive because they affect the same places in the brain as the street drug heroin. Take them exactly as prescribed and only under your doctor's close supervision.

Dollars&Sense
6 myth-busting truths about generic drugs

You can save up to 70 percent by choosing generic drugs, but are they as good or as safe as brand-name drugs? Here is what you need to know to separate fiction from fact.

Myth: Generics are not as safe as brand names.

Truth: Generic drugs must meet the same FDA safety standards as their brand-name equivalents. In fact, *Consumer Reports* and health watchdog *Public Citizen* say some generics may be safer than new brand-name drugs prescribed for the same condition. Here's why. From time to time, a few health dangers of a new drug are not discovered before FDA approval. But such problems are usually found before the drug is old enough to be available as a generic. Consequently, generic drugs are less likely to be pulled off the market or have extra warnings and restrictions added to their labels for safety reasons.

Myth: Generics are not as good as brand names.

Truth: To win FDA approval, a generic drug must meet the same guidelines for quality, purity, strength, and effectiveness as its brand-name equivalent. It must also use the same active ingredients, act just as fast, and work the same way in your body. The only difference is generic drugs can include other fillers and inactive ingredients, and these may cause an allergic reaction in some people. If you find this happens, you will have to avoid drugs that contain the problem ingredient.

Myth: The lower price means corners were cut.

Truth: Generics are cheaper simply because their makers don't have all the costs associated with creating a new drug. Any drug company that patents a new drug is granted a period of time to earn back the millions spent to create and test that drug.

When the patent period ends, other companies can copy and sell the drug for less money than it took to create it. They pass along that savings to you.

Myth: Brand-name drug costs don't rise much.

Truth: AARP reports that prices of brand-name drugs have been rising faster than inflation — sometimes twice as fast. Yet generic prices have lagged well behind inflation. For instance, thanks to a Walmart program, you may pay the low price of $4 for a month's supply of many generic drugs. Ask about this program at your local Walmart pharmacy.

Myth: Canadian drugs are cheaper than generics.

Truth: The seven best-selling generic drugs for chronic conditions in the United States are also available in Canada, so the FDA compared the costs. For five of the drugs, you would save by choosing the American generics instead of their Canadian brand name or generic versions.

Myth: All drugs have generic equivalents.

Truth: Some drugs are too new to have generic equivalents, but you might still find a generic drug with these tips.

▸ Ask both your doctor and pharmacist if your prescription has a generic equivalent. Your pharmacist may know about a generic drug that your doctor doesn't. If so, the pharmacist can consult with your doctor about changing your prescription.

▸ If your drug has no generic, ask your doctor if there are similar medications you can take that do have generic versions.

▸ Keep checking. Patent periods end every year, so many new generics will soon be on the shelves.

BPH

Top healers and helpers for enlarged prostate

For most men, the prostate gland gets larger with age, a condition known as benign prostatic hyperplasia (BPH). About 50 percent of men ages 51 to 60 have enlarged prostates, and almost 90 percent over age 80.

BPH is not cancerous, but it can certainly crimp your lifestyle. Enlarged prostates put the squeeze on your urethra, the tube carrying urine from the bladder out of the body. Men with BPH may have trouble urinating; feel the need to urinate often, especially at night; develop urinary tract infections; or become incontinent.

Fortunately, not all men with BPH have symptoms. In fact, doctors only recommend you seek treatment if symptoms become bothersome, or if you get frequent urinary tract infections. Luckily, men with this condition have lots of options.

When 'watchful waiting' makes good sense

Having BPH doesn't doom you to a life of expensive medication or surgeries. In fact, many men live fulfilling lives without any treatment. Experts call this approach "watchful waiting." It involves lifestyle changes to boost prostate health and an annual exam — and it could be right for you.

Benign prostatic hyperplasia can cause annoying urination problems, but rarely does it lead to serious complications, like kidney damage. Whether you choose to take medication, undergo surgery, or do nothing and wait mostly depends on the severity of your symptoms and how much they affect your life.

To gauge your symptoms, your doctor will examine you and ask a set of questions called the International Prostate Symptoms Score (IPSS) questionnaire. Your answers will help you and your doctor decide whether to choose watchful waiting, medication, surgery, or another procedure.

IPSS score	Rating	Treatment options
0 – 7	Mild	Consider watchful waiting if unbothered by minor symptoms, even if prostate is enlarged. Roughly 15 percent of "waiters" eventually need treatment.
8 – 19	Moderate	Decide whether symptoms are bothersome enough to merit treatment. Weigh complications, side effects, and cost against severity of symptoms.
20 – 35	Severe	Will most likely need medication or surgery.

Men who choose watchful waiting can take active steps to ease their symptoms and prevent them from getting worse.

▸ **Make it through the night.** Stop drinking fluids at 7 p.m. to cut down on nighttime bathroom trips.

▸ **Seize the opportunity.** Visit a restroom whenever you can, even if you don't feel the urge to go.

▸ **Cut out caffeine, especially coffee.** It's linked to a higher risk of BPH.

- **Limit alcohol.** Heavy drinking can aggravate your lower urinary tract.

- **Be choosy when picking a seat.** Take an aisle seat on airplanes, in theaters, and during other events.

- **Keep warm.** Cold weather improves muscle tone within the prostate, putting a stronger squeeze on your urinary tract and worsening common BPH symptoms.

- **Stay active.** Being immobile worsens urinary retention, while moderate exercise reduces urinary tract problems.

- **Say "no" to Sudafed.** Cold remedies that contain decongestants like pseudoephedrine can keep the muscles in your prostate and bladder from relaxing, making it more difficult to urinate.

- **Avoid allergy drugs.** Antihistamines, such as diphenhydramine (Benadryl), can slow urine flow in some men with BPH.

- **Be smart about diuretics.** They increase urination, a problem for men with BPH. Yet, they can also save your life if you have high blood pressure, so don't stop using them without your doctor's permission.

The latest scoop on saw palmetto

Millions of Americans take saw palmetto supplements, and European doctors routinely prescribe it for BPH. But does it really work? New studies raise questions and shed doubt on this popular herbal remedy.

European researchers analyzed the results of 17 studies on Permixon, a high-quality saw palmetto supplement for BPH. Overall, results were similar to those with alpha-blockers, the most common drugs for BPH. Permixon improved men's IPSS nearly five points, and it eased urinary problems in every study. Another analysis of 21 studies involving more than 3,000 men with BPH found saw palmetto supplements were about as effective as the

BPH drug finasteride (Proscar) and caused fewer side effects, such as erectile dysfunction.

But experts have never whole-heartedly endorsed this herb. They point out that most trials have included too few people, didn't last long enough, and had no standard measure for success.

To better test this popular supplement, researchers at the University of California conducted a randomized, placebo-controlled, double-blind trial — the "gold standard" of clinical studies. Out of 225 men with moderate to severe BPH, some took 160 milligrams (mg) of saw palmetto twice a day, and some took a placebo, or fake pill. After one year of treatment, the herb showed no more effect than the fake pills on urine flow, prostate size, ability to empty the bladder, or the men's quality of life.

If you decide to try saw palmetto, look for high-quality supplements, like those shown to work in clinical trials. You'll need an extract containing at least 85 percent fatty acids and 0.2 percent sterols. A standard dose would be 160 milligrams twice a day. Saw palmetto may keep your blood from clotting properly, so tell your doctor if you take it. If your symptoms don't improve in two months, stop taking the supplement.

More options for BPH sufferers

As many as one-third of men with BPH who decide to watch and wait choose to take supplements, such as saw palmetto. But other herbs and extracts are making news these days, too, for their potential to boost prostate health. Talk to your doctor about whether these therapies could be right for you.

Beta-sitosterol. Several studies suggest this mixture of plant compounds improves urine flow and other BPH symptoms, but it may also lead to erectile dysfunction and decreased sex drive. Some beta-sitosterol supplements are made to lower cholesterol. Be sure to buy those specifically made for BPH — the dosages and instructions differ greatly. Look for a brand that lists the specific amount of beta-sitosterol it contains, not just the total sterols, and take it on an empty stomach.

Stinging nettle. The root, not the leaves, of this prickly weed may put an end to enlarged prostates. Extracts made from stinging nettle roots also pack the steroid beta-sitosterol. Try the powdered root as a tea three to four times daily, or as a supplement. Experts typically suggest 4 to 6 grams of dried root daily for BPH.

Red clover. This common weed could one day prevent BPH and even prostate cancer. Two recent lab experiments found feeding mice a diet supplemented with red clover extract prevented the out-of-control growth of prostate cells that marks both BPH and prostate cancer. Scientists think compounds in red clover called isoflavones could be the key. If you decide to try red clover isoflavone supplements, take half the daily dose in the morning and half in the evening. Taking it with food rich in carbohydrates, like bread, beans, pasta, or potatoes, may help you absorb more isoflavones.

These nutritional superstars help you go with the flow

Do you wake up every few hours to take a trip to the bathroom? A poor diet can make your BPH symptoms worse. Fortunately, these two foods may keep those nightly bathroom visits at bay.

Tuck into tomatoes to crush your risk. Who doesn't love the summer? This season brings sunny days, warm weather, and — best of all — ripe and juicy tomatoes fresh from the garden.

But tomatoes are more than a tasty addition to your salads. It turns out that the chemical compound that gives tomatoes their red color — a nutrient called lycopene — could help lower your risk of BPH.

Italian scientists sorted men with enlarged prostates into two groups. All of them had lower urinary tract symptoms caused by their condition. One group took a daily placebo, while the other took a supplement containing lycopene and other nutrients each day. After three months, the men who took the supplement showed signs that their prostate growth had slowed.

Get your greens to fight off infections. Chinese researchers who tracked the eating habits of elderly men for four years discovered that a diet rich in fruit and vegetables was linked to a lower risk of BPH. Dark and leafy greens offered up the most protection. Experts say these veggies are packed with nutrients — like vitamin C and beta carotene — that combat inflammation and oxidative damage.

The men in the study who saw the most benefits ate sufficient amounts of fruits and vegetables, including around 100 grams of dark and leafy veggies a day. You can get more than half of that in 2 cups of raw spinach.

Need an excuse to crack open a can of sardines?

These flavorful fish are packed with protein. A small tin of sardines provides nearly half of the protein you need each day. Researchers say eating more of this nutrient may lower your risk of an enlarged prostate.

2 ways pepitas ward off prostate problems

Peter, Peter, pumpkin eater. Why was ol' Pete so fond of pumpkins? Perhaps he knew the seeds, often called pepitas, are packed with two ingredients that may protect his prostate.

Fix your flow with a natural plant compound. Frequent visits to the restroom. Inability to empty your bladder completely. Difficulty starting urination. Sound familiar? These are all symptoms of benign prostatic hyperplasia, or prostate enlargement. But how can you put the stream situation to rest? Beta-sitosterol.

This cholesterol-like compound is found in plant foods like pumpkin seeds. A review of four studies found it significantly improves the stop-and-go traffic of urinary flow, so you can empty out completely during your first trip to the loo.

You may get similar benefits from pumpkin seed oil. It can be pricey, but studies show it too can help urinary woes. Culinary experts suggest you use it in its raw form, rather than heated, to preserve nutrients. Try it whisked into vinaigrettes, drizzled over bread, or mixed into smoothies.

Manly mineral shrinks your prostate. The walnut-size prostate gland houses more zinc than most other organs. And for a good reason — the mineral is essential to prostate health. Experts say zinc may reduce the size of the prostate, relieving bothersome symptoms naturally.

Make sure you get the recommended 15 milligrams (mg) of zinc daily. An ounce of hulled pumpkin seeds will give you 2.1 mg. That's 14 percent of the amount of zinc you need each day, all packed into a crunchy little snack.

Walk away from BPH

If you want to reduce your risk of developing BPH, a brisk walk a few times around the block could help. A recent study found that active men were 25 percent less likely to have moderate to severe symptoms of the disorder or to have had surgery for BPH than less active men. Walking just two to three hours a week was enough exercise to bring about this level of risk reduction, but adding another three hours of walking per week reduced risk by another 10 percent.

Another reason to exercise is to keep off excess weight. According to a five-year study of more than 25,000 men, being 35 pounds or more overweight or gaining more than seven inches in your waist increases your risk of BPH by 75 percent after age 50. In fact, by age 75 to 80, about half the men with a waist size larger than 43 inches had moderate to severe urinary problems, with some of them even requiring surgery. On the other hand, only about one-third of the men with a waist size of 35 inches or less had significant urinary difficulties.

Practice Kegel exercises to strengthen your sphincter

The sphincter is a ring of muscle that opens and closes to allow urine to escape from the bladder. Keeping this muscle taut with exercises known as Kegels can help prevent involuntary leakage. Kegels were originally developed to help women through pregnancy, but they work just as effectively in helping men with BPH.

Because the muscle you are exercising is internal, it can be difficult to isolate. The easiest way to learn how to perform Kegels is while urinating. Here's how. As soon as urine starts to flow make a contraction to slow flow. Hold for 10 seconds. Then make another contraction to stop. Hold for another 10 seconds. Repeat until you're finished.

Get a definite diagnosis from your doctor before self-treating with saw palmetto or other supplements. Serious conditions such as prostate cancer can cause symptoms similar to BPH.

Do Kegels while you're urinating only as practice. Kegels are not intended to be performed while going to the bathroom, as doing so can eventually weaken the muscle.

Once you get the feel for it, you can exercise your sphincter when it's at rest. Kegels can be done anywhere – while you're driving, when you're sitting at your desk working, or when relaxing in the evening watching television. Perform the exercise by doing 10 to 15 contractions three to five times a day.

Ditch the decaf to dodge erectile dysfunction

Cutting back on your morning cup of coffee may be a good idea if you have BPH. Caffeine, after all, increases your need to urinate. And that's bad news if your enlarged prostate is blocking the flow of urine from your bladder.

But you might think twice before switching to decaf. Researchers studied the coffee-drinking habits of more than 21,400 men. They found that those who had 4 or more cups of decaffeinated coffee per day had a 37 percent greater risk of erectile dysfunction than those who didn't drink it.

Experts aren't quite sure why that's the case. They say that micronutients and antioxidants might somehow get removed during decaffeination. Another possibility? Harmful chemicals might be added during the process.

Cancer

Natural strategies to combat cancer

A few simple changes can improve your chances of staying healthy and cancer free, and all without drugs. The American Cancer Society says following these simple guidelines could prevent almost half of all cancer deaths.

▸ Stop smoking.

▸ Eat at least five servings total of fruits and vegetables every day.

▸ Buy foods made with whole grains instead of refined grains and sugar.

▸ Choose low-calorie, filling foods to maintain a healthy weight.

▸ Get moderate exercise 30 minutes a day, five days a week.

▸ Limit the red and processed meats you eat.

▸ Go in for regular cancer screenings.

The next few pages give you insider tips to ward off cancer, catch it early, and dodge the side effects of painful treatments.

Drink your way to better health

What is in your cup could help decide whether or not you develop cancer. Best of all, you probably enjoy some of these everyday beverages already. If not, maybe it's time to start. So raise your glass to the latest research, and toast to longer life.

Fight back with this brew. Tea, red wine, soybeans, fruits, and vegetables are loaded with flavonoids, a class of cancer-fighting compounds with anti-inflammatory and antioxidant powers. Out of 66,000 women in the Nurses' Health Study, those who got the most kaempferol, a flavonoid found mostly in tea, broccoli, and kale, sliced their chance of ovarian cancer nearly 40 percent. Experts say four daily cups of black or green tea, or two cups of broccoli, pack enough kaempferol to drop your risk, too.

Another study of 3,000 women living in Long Island found the flavonoids in tea, tomatoes, green salad, and apples lowered the boom on breast cancer risk in post-menopausal women as much as 46 percent. Other research suggests green tea, in particular, could help prevent invasive prostate cancer as well as gallbladder, colon, stomach, pancreatic, and esophageal cancers.

'Mooove' in on cancer. Getting more low-fat dairy in your diet could crush your risk of breast cancer. That's the finding from

Don't buy into deadly 'cure'

Scam artists claim that super-strong, 35-percent hydrogen peroxide can treat cancer, emphysema, AIDS, and other deadly illnesses. Don't be fooled. The Food and Drug Administration (FDA) has never approved high-strength hydrogen peroxide for internal use, and absolutely no research backs its curative claims. Even handling it is dangerous.

High-strength hydrogen peroxide is 10 times stronger — and more corrosive — than the over-the-counter kind used to clean wounds. Drinking it can irritate the stomach lining and cause ulcers. Taking it intravenously can inflame blood vessels, create gas bubbles in the blood, and lead to deadly allergic reactions.

a nine-year study of more than 68,000 women. Women who ate at least two servings of dairy a day — including milk, yogurt, and cheese — were 19 percent less likely to develop breast cancer after menopause. Likewise, women who got the most calcium in their daily diet, at least 1,250 mg, dropped their risk 20 percent. Supplements of calcium and vitamin D, however, didn't do the trick in this study.

Dairy may be just as important for men. In a new Swedish study, men who got the most calcium from food significantly cut their risk of colon and rectal cancers. Those who ate seven or more servings of dairy daily slashed their risk in half compared to men eating less than two servings a day.

Calcium may be just one of the protective ingredients. Dairy foods also contain conjugated linoleic acid, sphingolipids, and milk proteins, which are all linked to lower rates of colon cancer in animal studies. Milk by far packed the most preventive power, but hard cheese, sour cream, and regular cream also seemed to lower colon cancer risk. Discuss these results with your doctor before making big changes in your diet, though — some research links high-calcium diets to increased risk for advanced prostate cancer.

Wake up to a lower risk. That cup of joe could give you even more reason to get up in the morning. Among 90,000 Japanese, those who drank coffee every day had half the risk of liver cancer as people who rarely drank coffee — and the more cups, the lower their risk. A Canadian study, on the other hand, found coffee drinkers with BRCA gene mutations slashed their breast cancer risk as much as 70 percent. Again, the more cups they drank a day, the better. The caffeine in coffee may offer protection, but this wake-up brew is also packed with antioxidants — potential cancer-fighting compounds that may squash the development of tumors.

Enjoy an exotic juice. Drinking just 8 ounces of pure pomegranate juice a day could slow the growth of prostate cancer and curb the need for drastic treatments like hormone therapy or chemotherapy. Researchers at the University of California tested the juice on 46 men with prostate cancer. In four out of five men, PSA levels — a marker of prostate cancer progression — remained stable up to 4 1/2 years, nearly four times longer than normal. Men in this study drank the POM Wonderful brand of juice sold in supermarkets, but you can also make your own. Simply roll a pomegranate on the counter to soften it, poke a hole in the top, insert a straw, and drink to your health.

Sip this sweet treat. An extract made from store-bought apple juice stopped the growth of colon cancer cells in the lab. Scientists suspect the juice's healing powers belong to two antioxidants — proanthocyanidins and quercetin. However, a man-made extract of these compounds didn't work nearly as well as the whole juice in halting the growth of cancer cells, leading experts to believe apples may hold more mysterious cancer-fighters.

7 food secrets to sidestep cancer

Load your diet with these tasty foods, and you'll lower your risk of many types of cancer, including breast, prostate, colon, and lung cancers.

Start off with oatmeal. The soluble fiber in oatmeal is famous for banishing colon cancer, not to mention lowering cholesterol. Count on beans, oats, and many fruits and vegetables for this special fiber.

Turn it up with turmeric. Add a dash of curry to your next stir-fry. It's made with turmeric, a sizzling spice that may help prevent nine different cancers — prostate, breast, colon, skin, liver, stomach, mouth, blood, and lung. Topping cruciferous vegetables with turmeric could even fight existing prostate cancer.

Eat more legumes. If you eat beans or lentils less than once a month, you could be cheating yourself out of some hefty cancer protection. Studies have shown that eating these tasty legumes twice a week could lower your breast cancer risk 24 percent and help fend off colon, lung, and prostate cancers. A compound in legumes known as inositol pentakisphosphate may stop cancer cells from growing and could boost the effectiveness of anti-cancer drugs.

Savor tasty tomatoes. Thanks to whopping amounts of lycopene, tomatoes are potent against prostate and pancreatic cancers. Cook them in olive oil to double the lycopene you absorb, and eat cooked tomato products like sauces, which pack more lycopene than raw tomatoes.

Pour on olive oil. It's full of healthy fats, one of which — oleic acid — targets the gene that promotes breast cancer, while other compounds called phenols protect against colon cancer.

Pick a pail of berries. Berries pack a three-part punch against cancer. Studies have shown that blueberries keep colon cancer cells from growing; the ellagic acid in raspberries and strawberries kills cervical cancer cells; and cranberry juice seems to stop cancer from spreading throughout the body.

Go nuts for selenium. Selenium-rich foods could help prevent cancer of the colon, rectum, stomach, esophagus, and lung. Just six to eight Brazil nuts give you 543 micrograms of selenium, nearly 10 times the amount you need each day.

Highly salted foods are some of the most dangerous for your bowel, because they are associated with a greater risk of stomach cancer. Don't overindulge in pickled items for this reason. One exception — miso soup. The soy in it seems to cancel out the harmful effects of its salt.

Crunch down on cancer with crucifers

If Superman were a food, he'd be a cruciferous vegetable. Crunchy munchies like broccoli, cabbage, cauliflower, and watercress really know how to knock out cancer.

Cruciferous vegetables contain large amounts of glucosinolates (GLS). When you chew, chop, or otherwise prepare these veggies, the GLS break down into potent cancer-fighting chemicals including isothiocyanates (ITCs) and indoles. These compounds have been shown to prevent and slow the development of cancer in lab and animal experiments.

One type of ITC known as phenethyl-ITC (PEITC) and sulforaphane, a compound found in broccoli, seem especially promising. Experts think eating vegetables rich in these compounds could help prevent cancer as well as slow the growth of existing tumors, even in people genetically prone to certain cancers. So if you want to cut your risk of cancer and avoid drugs and surgery, give a helping hand to your immune system with these delicious foods.

Beat the odds of breast cancer. The BRCA gene makes two proteins, BRCA1 and BRCA2, that repair damaged DNA. People with a faulty BRCA gene have a harder time repairing DNA and, as a result, face a greater risk of certain cancers, including breast, ovarian, and prostate. Lucky for them, an indole known as indole-3-carinol (I3C) in broccoli, cauliflower, and cabbage boosts levels of BRCA repair proteins. These three vegetables seem to be particularly potent against breast cancer.

▸ Italian researchers discovered that juice squeezed from cauliflower leaves prevented the growth of both estrogen (ER)-positive and ER-negative breast cancer cells. Lightly cook or eat cauliflower raw, since cooking destroys most of the anticancer compounds.

▸ In Europe, Polish women tend to face low rates of this disease, so researchers compared Polish natives to Polish-American immigrants. The women who ate three or more servings of raw or lightly cooked cabbage each week during their teenage years reaped a powerful benefit. Their breast cancer risk was a staggering 72 percent less than women who had eaten fewer than 1.5 servings weekly.

▸ A new lab study finds sulforaphane, broccoli's powerful anti-cancer compound, may not only help prevent the mutations that turn normal cells cancerous, it also keeps existing breast cancer cells from growing and spreading.

Put the squeeze on prostate cancer. Eating cruciferous vegetables, especially broccoli, at least twice a month could cut your risk of prostate cancer, say researchers at Mt. Sinai School of Medicine in New York. In a related lab experiment, mice with

Supplements sabotage cancer therapy

Cancer patients often take antioxidant supplements like vitamin C alongside regular radiation or chemotherapy. Unfortunately, popping antioxidant pills could actually sabotage these treatments.

Radiation and chemotherapy kill cancer cells by creating free radicals — the same compounds antioxidants disarm. Plus, cancer cells absorb more vitamin C than healthy cells, boosting their defenses against treatment. At least one study found women with breast cancer who took antioxidant vitamins and minerals alongside standard cancer treatment had lower survival rates than women who opted for standard therapy alone.

While eating antioxidant-rich foods could help prevent this disease, numerous clinical trials show supplements do not and may, in fact, raise some people's cancer risk. Save your money and stick with natural food sources.

prostate cancer that ate a small amount of PEITC daily for a month had half as many tumors as those that didn't get the extract. How many greens does that mean? A single ounce of watercress yields five times the amount of PEITC needed to slow the growth of prostate tumors in these mice. Serve up a side and dig in.

Lower your risk of lung cancer. What's more, animal research shows PEITC and sulforaphane could help prevent lung cancer in smokers and former smokers. And a study recently published in *The Lancet* found non-smokers who ate cabbage or a combination of broccoli and brussels sprouts at least once a week enjoyed the lowest risk for lung cancer, thanks to those famous isothiocyanates.

5 great reasons you should fuel up on fiber today

Your future could be brighter — just by making a simple change in the way you eat. New research suggests fiber doesn't just fight colon cancer and help keep you regular. Eating more fiber can help prevent at least five kinds of cancer. Here are a few things you probably didn't know.

Fend off deadly cancer of the esophagus with popcorn? Want a good reason to choose fiber-packed, air-popped popcorn instead of baked potato chips? According to Irish research, people who eat the most fiber have less risk of esophageal cancer. Experts suspect fiber's power to help control weight and improve gastroesophageal reflux (GERD) may help keep you cancer-free.

Scary link between refined grains and kidney cancer. People who eat the most refined grains raise their risk of kidney cancer with every bite. Refined grains include foods like low-fiber white bread and baked goods. Fortunately, people who consume the most fiber may reduce their risk of kidney cancer by 15 to 20 percent.

Whole grains; legumes like peas, beans, lentils, and peanuts; and cruciferous veggies like cabbage and broccoli may be particularly good protectors.

Experts suggest fiber may safeguard your kidneys by reducing the amount of toxins kidneys must process and helping prevent obesity. Fermentation of fiber in your gut also generates compounds that promote anti-inflammatory and anticancer activities throughout your body.

> Often sold as an herbal treatment for cancer, bitter apricot kernels produce cyanide and can be poisonous at high doses.

Shut out prostate cancer with a peanut butter sandwich. Aim for 38 grams of fiber a day if you're a man. A European study of more than 3,000 men showed that those who ate more fiber had less danger of prostate cancer over the next 12 years — especially if they ate lots of insoluble fiber and legumes. For something quick and delicious, try natural peanut butter on whole-grain toast.

Cut stomach cancer risk with just 10 extra grams of fiber every day. This small change in your diet may lower your odds of stomach cancer by 44 percent, Chinese researchers report. If you add more fiber, increase your daily amount gradually over time, or you may experience gas and bloating.

Learn to love fruits, veggies, and whole-grains to evade breast cancer. A British review of research found that women who eat the most fiber have less risk of breast cancer than women who eat the least. Researchers suspect fiber may help block breast cancer by controlling estrogen and blood sugar levels. For best results, women should aim for 25 grams of fiber every day.

Liquid gold takes the sting out of cancer treatments

An explosion of lifesaving cancer therapies bring new hope, but, in many cases, also new side effects. Enter honey. Evidence shows it can help heal some damage caused by radiation and chemotherapy.

Dermatitis. Radiation harms skin cells, which can leave you with itchy, red, and painful dermatitis. In separate studies, women undergoing radiation for breast cancer:

▸ had less severe dermatitis if they applied manuka honey to their skin twice a day, beginning the first day of radiation.

▸ found honey-infused gauze eased pain, itching, and irritation, and helped skin heal faster after radiation.

Talk to your doctor about using medical-grade, manuka-infused ointments and bandages such as products marketed under the brand name MEDIHONEY.

Mucositis. Chemotherapy and radiation may kill cancer cells, but they also kill the benign cells lining your mouth, throat, and digestive tract. The result is mucositis — painful ulcers that can make it hard to eat, drink, or simply swallow.

Multiple studies show that eating honey can help prevent mucositis in people getting radiation for head and neck cancer. Most found relief by taking four teaspoons of honey three times a day throughout the course of their treatment. To try it yourself, swish each mouthful for up to two minutes, then slowly swallow it. You can use manuka honey, but you don't have to. Many types will work.

Vitamin D in food and supplements is measured in either IU (international units) or micrograms of calciferol. One microgram equals 40 IU.

In a surprising twist, researchers recently stumbled upon an unexpected benefit from a honey and coffee combination.

They found a homemade brew healed chemo-induced mucositis better than steroids and better than honey mixed with water. Discuss this remedy with your doctor before you try it.

▸ Brew strong coffee made from 10 ounces of water with about six tablespoons of instant coffee.

▸ Stir in about one cup of local or manuka honey.

▸ Sip then swallow three teaspoons of this mixture every three hours for one week.

Since heat destroys some of the healing properties of honey, let your coffee cool to room temperature before adding the honey.

Cut cancer risk without spending a dime

Skip the supplements and save your money by taking advantage of the cheapest medicine on earth. Read on for these life-saving, cancer-busting secrets.

Get up and get moving. You don't have to be a fitness fanatic, but you do need some exercise every day. Although it won't guarantee you a cancer-free life, it just might help you beat the odds.

▸ Australian researchers found that moderate exercise protected against prostate cancer, while Harvard scientists discovered regular, vigorous exercise slowed the progression of prostate cancer in men over 65.

▸ Lab studies show exercise can prevent the development of skin cancer and slow the growth of existing skin tumors in mice.

▸ A Canadian study links recreational activity with a drop in ovarian cancer rates in both pre- and postmenopausal women. The more exercise, the lower their risk. Being sedentary more than six hours daily may boost women's risk.

▸ Overweight women who start exercising could significantly drop their breast cancer risk. Scientists believe the amount of fat in your body influences the amount of estrogen in your system. High levels of estrogen in postmenopausal women point to increased risk of breast cancer. Based on a recent study, exercising moderately 45 minutes a day, five days a week can help you lose enough fat to lower estrogen levels and slice cancer risk. But dieting isn't enough. Women who dropped pounds but did not exercise actually saw their estrogen levels rise over the course of a year.

Learn to relax. Experts suspect chronic stress suppresses the immune system and affects cells' ability to repair damage, which can set the stage for some cancers. Johns Hopkins researchers put an unlucky group of mice under constant stress. The results — compared to relaxed mice, the stressed-out mice were five times more likely to get skin cancer, and their cancers developed nearly three times faster.

These experts suggest people at high risk of skin cancer consider taking classes in stress reduction, but you could manage without spending money. You'll get a good laugh out of this easy way to relieve pain, lower stress, and boost immunity. Researchers have learned laughter can fight the immune-suppressing effects of stress. Women who laughed out loud at a funny video gave a big boost to their immune system. Simply watching a humorous show didn't do the trick, though — only women who laughed aloud saw a benefit.

Stop smoking. Smoking contributes to up to 90 percent of lung cancer deaths. Compared to those who don't smoke, men smokers are 23 times more likely to get lung cancer, while women smokers are 13 times more likely. Secondhand smoke is no better. According to a new Surgeon General's report, there are no safe levels of secondhand smoke. Breathing even small amounts at work or home increases your risk of lung cancer as much as 30 percent, plus boosts your risk of heart disease and heart attack.

Keep a lid on cholesterol. A history of high cholesterol or gallstones may increase your risk for prostate cancer. In fact, the earlier in life you develop high cholesterol, the greater your risk. Similarly, research shows overweight, postmenopausal women who have low levels of "good" HDL cholesterol have a higher risk of breast cancer.

Experts say low HDL can signal high levels of cancer-causing hormones including estrogen, androgens, and insulin. This might explain why some studies show cholesterol-lowering statin drugs seem to ward off prostate cancer. The jury is still out on this protective effect. In the meantime, follow your doctor's orders and check the *High cholesterol* chapter for advice on keeping these important numbers under control.

Count on friends. Making time for friends and family could help you survive ovarian cancer. Researchers found women with the disease who had a strong social support system also had lower levels of IL-6, a pro-inflammatory compound linked to the spread of ovarian cancer. Don't wait until illness strikes to reach out to loved ones. Strengthen the bonds of friendships and family, and you just might live a lot longer.

Beware: Laxative can harm kidneys

The FDA warns that oral sodium phosphate (OSP) solutions (Visicol, OsmoPrep) used to flush out bowels before a colonoscopy can lead to kidney failure in some people. Ask your doctor to prescribe a non-sodium phosphate laxative before a colonoscopy if you are on a low-salt diet, use diuretics, take drugs for high blood pressure or arthritis, or have a history of kidney problems. Also, tell your doctor if you have taken a laxative for constipation in the last week.

Beat disease with fun in the sun

Everyone knows too much time in the sun can cause cancer, but — surprise — so can too little. Your skin turns sunlight into vitamin D, and new studies link vitamin D deficiencies to 13 different cancers, including prostate, colon, breast, and ovarian.

Ultraviolet B (UVB) rays from the sun react with a compound in skin to produce vitamin D. The liver and kidneys process this vitamin but so do cells in other parts of the body, such as the prostate and colon. In these areas, vitamin D stops cancer cells from multiplying and spreading and triggers them to self-destruct.

Many new studies link high levels of D in the blood with a drop in cancer risk. One study found people who got the equivalent of 1500 International Units (IU) of this vitamin daily slashed their risk of getting any cancer by 17 percent and were a whopping 45 percent less likely to die from digestive cancers.

Unfortunately, vitamin D deficiency increases your risk, and it is amazingly common. People who live in the northeastern United States, dark-skinned people, and seniors all face a potential shortage.

▸ People in the Northeast don't get enough UVB rays from November through March to make vitamin D.

▸ The pigment melanin in skin acts like a sunscreen, so darker-skinned people absorb less UVB and make less vitamin D than lighter-skinned people. In fact, one survey found 42 percent of Black women were deficient.

▸ Everyone absorbs less vitamin D with age, so older adults need even more of it.

The National Academy of Sciences recommends people ages 51 to 70 get 600 IU daily, and seniors over 70 get 800 IU daily. But

other experts say that's not enough to fight cancer or prevent deficiencies, especially in northeastern areas. Some experts suggest
aiming for 1,000 IU of vitamin D each day.

In most parts of the United States, that means a stroll with the
sun on your neck, shoulders, and back (without sunscreen) each day
between 11 a.m. and 2 p.m. — 15 minutes a day in summer and 20
minutes a day in early fall and late spring. Black people need twice as
much sun. Other experts, including dermatologists, argue inexpensive vitamin D supplements are the safest way to boost blood levels.

Discuss your options with your doctor and ask how much of this
nutrient he thinks you need based on your age, location, and skin
tone. Then follow these tips to get the "sunshine vitamin" safely.

▸ Avoid burning. The same UVB rays that make vitamin D also
cause skin cancer. Limit your sun exposure to 20 minutes a day
if you burn easily and tan poorly. More than that will not
noticeably increase your D levels.

▸ Hold off showering, bathing, or swimming for an hour after
being in the sun to give your body time to absorb the vitamin.

▸ Get your daily D from supplements if you have fair skin, are sensitive to sunlight, or take medications that cause light sensitivity.

▸ Shop for cereals, milk, butter, and margarine fortified with
vitamin D.

▸ Angle to occasionally eat fatty, coldwater fish such as tuna, sardines, herring, and mackerel, all rich in this nutrient.

▸ Discuss vitamin D supplements with your doctor first if you take
calcium-channel blockers or thiazide diuretics.

▸ Avoid getting more than 2,000 IU of vitamin D from food and
supplements in a single day.

Vitamin offers new hope for cancer

Decades ago, two-time Nobel prize winner Linus Pauling reported that high doses of vitamin C could cure cancer. Mayo Clinic studies found no such benefit, and doctors stopped pursuing it. Now, new evidence suggests he could have been right.

In Pauling's studies, people with cancer took vitamin C by mouth as well as intravenously (IV). However, in the Mayo Clinic studies that followed, people only took it by mouth. Experts now think IV treatments hold the key.

Getting it through an IV raises blood levels of vitamin C 25 times higher than taking the same dose by mouth. Concentrated C is toxic to cancer cells but not to normal, healthy tissue. Once it reaches the tumor, this super-dose of vitamin C reacts with other fluids to create hydrogen peroxide, which seems to kill cancerous cells. Scientists say it's impossible to get enough vitamin C by mouth to raise blood levels high enough to produce hydrogen peroxide.

Three recent case studies in a prominent medical journal make a strong case for this old treatment. Three people each with different types of cancer got high doses of vitamin C by IV weekly and monthly for up to four years. Each person saw their tumors shrink and the cancer enter remission.

All three people took other nutritional supplements in addition to the vitamin C, and two of the three underwent traditional therapy, such as surgery and radiation. Researchers say this could account for these miraculous "cures," but they still believe vitamin C played a strong role. Experts say it's too soon to tell cancer sufferers to seek IV vitamin-C treatments, but they believe enough evidence exists to warrant real clinical trials in people.

Even if it proves effective, this therapy probably will not work for all types of cancer, and not everyone is a candidate for high doses of vitamin C. Experts say people with renal failure, iron over-load, a history of oxalate kidney stones, or on dialysis should not try this treatment.

Cancer screening sparks controversy

Will you automatically agree to a cancer screening your doctor sug-gests? Should you worry about overscreening? False positives? You may hear a different philosophy depending on who you talk to — your insurance company, a cancer survivor, a consumer advocate, a statistician, or even a medical researcher.

The National Cancer Institute identifies four different kinds of screening tests. They were designed to help find cancer in its earliest stages — when it's easier to treat and often before you have any symptoms.

▸ Physical exam. Your doctor will check your body for any signs of disease, such as lumps, tenderness, or skin changes.

▸ Laboratory tests. Samples of your blood, urine, tissue, or other substances are sent to a lab where they look for chemical or bio-logical indicators of cancer.

▸ Imaging procedures. Detailed pictures of areas inside your body help doctors diagnose and plan treatment. Examples are X-rays, ultrasounds, magnetic resonance imaging (MRI), and computed tomography (CT) scans.

▸ Genetic tests. Some cancers, like breast cancer, are often linked to specific gene mutations.

Unfortunately, the guidelines on cancer screenings have become convoluted due, in part, to evolving technology. Tests have become more sensitive, detecting tiny potential cancers that often disap-pear on their own or end up being harmless.

Here's information on screenings for three major types of cancer. Just remember, only you can decide what is right for you.

Colon cancer. Affecting the lower part of your digestive system, colon cancer usually begins as small clumps of noncancerous cells called adenomatous polyps. In time, some of these polyps can become cancerous. You rarely have symptoms from colon polyps, which makes screening that much more important.

The U.S. Preventive Services Task Force (USPSTF) is an independent panel of medical experts who review screenings, counseling services, and preventive medications to make recommendations to doctors and patients. They say every 50-year-old should be screened for colon cancer by having either a colonoscopy, sigmoidoscopy, or fecal occult blood test but only until age 75. If you are at average risk of developing colon cancer, tests like these can cut your risk of developing late-stage cancer by 70 percent.

Breast cancer. The American Cancer Society recommends that mammograms for women start at age 40 and continue every year as long as you are in good health. There is recent debate, however, based on 50 years of research, over whether mammograms might do more harm than good. The concerns include overdiagnosis; overtreatment of benign tumors including surgery, chemotherapy, and radiation; increased risk of harmful side effects of that treatment; and no reduction in the number of advanced breast cancer cases.

Here are the new, and somewhat controversial, guidelines from the USPSTF:

- No routine screening mammography from ages 40 to 49 unless called for by individual circumstances.
- A mammogram every two years between the ages of 50 and 74.
- No clear evidence to either support or oppose mammograms for women over 74 years old.

Mammograms save lives, although many experts admit the screening has shortcomings. Until something better comes along, women need to understand the limitations and possible consequences so they can make informed decisions.

Prostate cancer. PSA is the acronym for prostate-specific antigen. This enzyme enters the bloodstream when there's something amiss in the prostate gland. It was an important discovery back in 1970 because the antigen tips off doctors that tumors are recurring in men who have been treated for prostate cancer. But in 1994, the U.S. Food and Drug Administration (FDA) approved the PSA test to screen for previously undetected prostate cancer. Doctors hastily embraced it as a simple, no-harm-done addition to the routine blood tests conducted during a man's annual physical examination.

Over the next two decades, the incidence of early-stage prostate cancer rose dramatically, while deaths from late-stage prostate disease took a dive. And, not surprisingly, nearly a million healthy men with elevated PSAs but no symptoms of disease were frightened into unnecessary radical surgery to have their prostates removed. This left the majority of them struggling with a lifetime of impotence and incontinence. As a result, the PSA test has become one of the hottest and most contentious medical controversies of modern times.

You may be surprised to learn the USPSTF recommends against PSA-based screening for men in generally good health, regardless of age. This recommendation, however, does not apply to men suspected of having prostate cancer.

Crucial questions you must ask your doctor

The National Institutes of Health and *Consumer Reports* recently examined the role cancer screening plays in today's health care. Their results may surprise you — too many people are getting tests they don't need, while too few are getting tests that could save their lives. Everyone should ask these six questions before undergoing any test.

1. What is my risk for cancer compared with the average person?

2. Does this test often give inaccurate results?

3. Can I choose a different test?

4. What should I do if the results are positive?

5. Are there any dangers or side effects?

6. What do I need to do to get ready for the test?

Also ask your doctor how much the test will cost, and how long it will take to get the results. All of this information will help you make the best choice for your health.

An aspirin a day keeps cancer at bay

More than 40 years ago, researchers discovered when blood loses its ability to clot, cancer cells cannot easily spread, or metastasize. Decades later, aspirin, one of the most widely used anti-clotting medications, is still under review as a safe, effective way to lower your risk of cancer.

The most convincing evidence concerns colon cancer. It's long been known that aspirin protects your colon by preventing the formation of intestinal polyps, which can turn into cancer. The question has always been how. One theory is that it blocks your body from creating prostaglandins, chemicals important to these precancerous growths. New studies suggest aspirin also causes mutated intestinal stem cells to die. The theory is, take a daily aspirin and you'll not only reduce your risk of developing colon cancer, but improve your chances of surviving it.

Here's even more compelling evidence that aspirin is a serious cancer-fighter.

▸ Women who take a daily aspirin could reduce their risk of ovarian cancer by 20 percent, compared to those who use aspirin less than once a week.

▸ Yale researchers say they have evidence the longer someone takes low-dose aspirin, the smaller their chances of developing pancreatic cancer. In studies, a 10-year aspirin habit cut this risk in half.

▸ The famous Women's Health Initiative, involving close to 60,000 women ages 50 to 79, reports aspirin protected against melanoma, the deadliest form of skin cancer, possibly by controlling inflammation.

▸ Barrett's esophagus is a precancerous condition usually linked to ongoing acid reflux and affecting the tube that carries food from your mouth to your stomach. Some people with Barrett's are more likely than others to have this condition turn into full-blown esophageal cancer. Aspirin may tip the odds in their favor by restricting cancer cell growth.

In addition, aspirin helps fight head, neck, throat, endometrial, and liver cancers.

A close look at all the current research leads experts to believe low-dose aspirin — anywhere from 75 to 325 milligrams daily — can give you some protection against various cancers if taken for at least five years. But because aspirin keeps your blood from clotting, it also raises your risk of dangerous bleeding and stroke. Ask your doctor if long-term aspirin therapy is right for you.

Shrink your cancer risk: 10 environmental toxins to avoid

Compounds found in everyday consumer products can be hazardous to your health. The Centers for Disease Control and Prevention (CDC) currently measures more than 300 environmental chemicals to see how much people are exposed to through air, water, food, soil, dust, or consumer products. This is called biomonitoring.

The list of potential hazards is full of unpronounceable words, like N,N-Diethyl-meta-toluamide, which you may know as DEET, an insect repellant first marketed in 1957 that can cause skin and neurological problems.

If you were to learn about each chemical, how it impacts human health, and where it can be found, you might book a seat on the first spaceship off the planet.

But don't give up hope. Despite the increasing number of chemicals introduced by manufacturers every year, governments are working to regulate their safety. Along with the CDC, other organizations like the National Toxicology Program, part of the U.S. Department of Health and Human Services; the Environmental Protection Agency (EPA); and the Food and Drug Administration (FDA) study, test, and promote safe levels of these environmental toxins.

Focus on the things you can control right now. Switch to non-toxic and natural alternatives for products you use on your body and in and around your home.

Bisphenol A (BPA). BPA is used in polycarbonate plastics, epoxy resins, and in certain thermal paper products, including some cash register and ATM receipts. To reduce your exposure to BPA, the National Toxicology Program offers these tips.

▸ Avoid plastic containers with #7 or the letters "PC" on the bottom.

- Stop microwaving food in polycarbonate plastic containers. Over time, the chemical can break down from the high temperatures.

- Wash polycarbonate plastic containers by hand. Avoid your dishwasher's harsh detergents.

- Eat fresh or frozen foods and rely less on canned foods.

- Choose glass, porcelain, or stainless steel containers, especially for hot food and liquids.

- Buy baby bottles and toys labeled BPA free.

Atrazine. This agricultural pesticide is widely used in the U.S. It's sometimes used on residential lawns, especially in Florida and the Southeast. Buy a water filter certified to remove atrazine from your drinking water, and choose organic fruits and vegetables.

Phthalates. These chemicals, often called plasticizers, are used to make plastics more flexible and harder to break. Avoid plastic food containers, children's toys, and plastic wrap made from PVC, which has the recycling label #3. Some soap, shampoo, hair spray, and nail polish also contain phthalates. Always read labels and avoid products that list added "fragrance." This general term sometimes means hidden phthalates.

Flame retardants. Added to furniture, clothing, building materials, and other products, these chemicals reduce the likelihood of fire. Ask before buying furniture if it contains flame retardant chemicals. Use a vacuum with a HEPA filter to cut down on toxic house dust. Take care when replacing old carpet since the padding underneath may contain toxins.

Arsenic. This highly poisonous element can cause bladder, lung, and skin cancer, and it may also cause kidney and liver cancer. It harms the central and peripheral nervous systems, as well as heart and blood vessels, and causes serious skin problems. It contaminates drinking water either from natural deposits in the earth or from industrial and agricultural pollution. Use a water filter that lowers arsenic levels.

Mercury. Methylmercury builds up in the tissues of fish, with larger and older fish usually having the highest levels. To limit your exposure, choose wild salmon and farmed trout.

Perfluorooctanoic acid (PFOA). This example of a perfluorochemical (PFC) is used on nonstick pans, as well as in stain and water-resistant coatings on clothing, furniture, and carpets.

Organophosphate pesticides. These pesticides affect the nervous system by disrupting the enzyme that regulates the neurotransmitter acetylcholine. Because some of these pesticides are very poisonous, avoid them by choosing organic produce.

Glycol ethers. You can be exposed to these through cleaning products, liquid soaps, and cosmetics. Avoid ingredients such as 2-butoxyethanol (EGBE), methoxydiglycol (DEGME), 2-methoxyethanol, and 2-ethoxyethanol.

Parabens. These chemicals are widely used as preservatives in cosmetics and personal care products, and as antimicrobials to prevent food spoilage. According to the European Commission's Scientific Committee on Consumer Products, some parabens can disrupt your endocrine system and cause reproductive and developmental disorders. Avoid these ingredients — methylparaben, propylparaben, butylparaben, or benzylparaben.

Dollars&Sense
Secret to saving up to 50 percent on drugs

Your prescription drug could be one of the few health items that qualifies for a two-for-one deal. The secret is pill splitting. You can buy twice the dosage you need for a few cents more, then split the pill in half for two cheaper doses. But be careful. Some people have experienced dangerous effects and overdoses from splitting the wrong pill or splitting improperly. It's important to know how to do it safely.

First of all, never use a knife. Research suggests you could swallow up to 20 percent more or less medicine than you need if a pill does not break perfectly in half. Low-cost drugstore pill splitters are your best option.

Avoid the possible problems and side effects of splitting pills by remembering these don'ts.

▸ Don't split capsules, extended-release tablets, enteric-coated pills, or pills containing more than one drug.

▸ Don't split pills without a score mark — the line on the pill that helps it break.

▸ Don't split a tablet if taking precisely the right dose is critical — as with warfarin.

▸ Don't split pills if you have poor vision, arthritis, or another problem that prevents precise splitting. Ask your pharmacist or someone else for help.

Studies suggest the following pills are safe to split and can save you up to 50 percent in prescription costs: atorvastatin (Lipitor), citalopram (Celexa), clonazepam (Klonopin), doxazosin (Cardura), lisinopril (Zestril), nefazodone (Serzone), olanzapine (Zyprexa), paroxetine (Paxil), pravastatin (Pravachol), sertraline (Zoloft), and sildenafil (Viagra). Ask your doctor and pharmacist about others.

Cataracts

Hold on to your sight — and your savings

Cataracts are responsible for 40 percent of all cases of blindness in the world. And more than half of all Americans develop this vision problem by age 80. In fact, Medicare spends $3.5 billion on cataract treatment every year — around $27 of taxpayer money for each household in the United States.

Cataracts occur when the lens in your eye starts clouding over, often turning your vision dimmer or blurrier. Cataract surgery can usually restore vision, but your best — and cheapest — bet is to prevent cataracts altogether. Experts suspect cataract surgeries might drop by half if people could slow their cataract development by just 10 years. This chapter shows you ways to prevent cataracts and tips to save money while doing it.

Watch out for top cataract-causing drugs

Keep your eye on this disturbing list of drugs that can lead to sight-stealing cataracts. The ones with an asterisk are the most likely troublemakers.

- ▸ *corticosteroids like prednisone
- ▸ *tamoxifen but not raloxifene
- ▸ *psoralens

- *glaucoma medicines including demecarium, isoflurophate, and echothiophate
- *antipsychotic medicines like chlorpromazine
- thyroid hormone
- potassium-sparing diuretics
- amiodarone
- tricyclic antidepressants

In addition, Zocor and Pravachol can make cataracts worse if you already have them.

Talk to your doctor if you take any of the medicines above. You may be able to switch to a drug that doesn't raise cataract risk — or possibly take other precautions.

4 ways to fight cataracts every day

You can lower your chances of developing cataracts by taking steps to avoid certain risk factors.

Go unleaded. Surprising new research shows that lead exposure can raise cataract odds. If the water pipes in your home are dull gray and can be scratched with a key, they may be tainting your water with lead. Either use a water filter that promises to remove lead, or get your water tested.

Think lean. Control your weight, and you'll help control your risk for cataracts. You may have even more to gain by losing pounds if you have diabetes, high blood pressure, glaucoma, or other eye diseases. All these conditions raise your cataract risk, too.

To absorb the most eye-saving lutein and zeaxanthin, add foods that have some fat. In a small study, people absorbed seven times as much lutein from a salad with avocado compared to a salad that was fat-free.

Quit and win. Research shows that heavy smokers and people who drink alcohol frequently have a higher chance of cataracts. Find ways to quit.

Say N-O to UV. Exposure to UV light from sunlight raises your risk of cataracts, but that doesn't mean you have to spend big bucks on designer sunglasses. In fact, testing shows that sunglasses under $10 can give you enough protection. The trick is to find the right ones.

▸ Look for labels that say "UV absorption up to 400nm," labels that promise to block 99 percent of UV, or shades with the Skin Cancer Foundation's Seal of Recommendation.

▸ Choose wraparound frames and lenses that are large enough to cover your eyes well.

▸ Don't assume that mirrored or polarized glasses block enough UV light. These features only block glare. A darker lens also doesn't affect the amount of UV light blocked.

Don't wait to buy sunglasses if yours don't offer adequate protection. But to get the best deal on a spare pair or a replacement, shop in August when bargains are more likely.

Save your sight with smart food choices

Eat six to 10 servings of fruits and vegetables every day, and you could cut your cataract risk by as much as 15 percent, according to a recent study. Emphasize foods like spinach, collards, tomato juice, and kale. They're high in the eye-saving carotenoids lutein and zeaxanthin.

Although eye damage from sunlight may help cause cataracts, these super nutrients may slash that damage by up to 60 percent.

Stick with whole foods. You can try lutein-zeaxanthin supplements, but most people get 2 milligrams (mg) per day from their diet already. It's not too difficult to eat the 6 mg daily associated with a reduced risk of cataracts. Just a half cup of cooked kale or spinach will supply that amount. Celery and broccoli are also good, convenient choices.

Some medicines — like cholesterol reducers — may blunt your ability to absorb lutein and zeaxanthin. Ask your doctor or pharmacist whether medicines you take affect absorption, and get his advice on what to do about it.

Choose fats wisely. A new research study suggests that women who eat the most omega-3 fish oils may have up to 12 percent less risk of cataracts than women who eat the least. But additional research found that those more prone to cataracts were the women who ate the most omega-6 fats from foods like mayonnaise, sunflower oil, safflower oil, and soybean oil.

Trim your carbs. U.S. Department of Agriculture research has found that you're more likely to get cataracts if you eat high amounts of carbohydrates — 200 grams or more — per day. Limit your carbohydrates by getting rid of junk foods like sweets and potato chips.

Other foods that may help fight cataracts include green and black tea, turmeric, and glutathione-rich foods like asparagus, avocado, and orange juice as well as quercetin-rich foods like onions.

Call on turmeric to spice up your sight

Your spice rack does more than zest up your dinner plate. If you know what to look for, you'll find potent protection against all sorts of ailments. And one exotic ingredient could hold the key to thwarting cataracts.

Turmeric — a golden spice from India — is loaded with a naturally occurring chemical called curcumin. And experts say this nutrient has some serious sight-saving powers.

Studies show it can fight off oxidative damage to your eye's lens. And it helps pump up the levels of vitamin C in your eyes as well, so you'll get a double dose of antioxidants.

Researchers haven't figured out how much turmeric you need to add to your diet to fight cataracts, but keep your eyes peeled for more information in the future.

In the meantime, sprinkle this exotic spice on roast veggies, stir it into your morning scrambled eggs, or add it to a smoothie. It's a good idea to add black or cayenne pepper to your turmeric, too. It will help your body absorb more sight-saving antioxidants.

Cheap, easy, and safe! Surprising way to protect your vision

Your aging eyes can suffer from a number of serious conditions, but an easy exercise like walking can help protect them. Research shows that regular aerobic exercise reduces your risk of developing cataracts, macular degeneration, and glaucoma.

For this benefit, walk briskly enough to get your heart pumping. If you can step it up, you'll reap even more protection.

▸ In recent studies, men who ran more than 5.7 miles a day slashed their cataract risk by more than one-third compared to men who ran less than 1.4 miles daily.

▶ For every 0.6 miles people ran every day, their chances of developing age-related macular degeneration (AMD) dropped 10 percent. Bump your average jog up to at least two miles a day and you've more than doubled your protection against AMD compared to running a mile or less.

▶ Ocular perfusion pressure (OPP) is the relationship between your whole body's blood pressure and the fluid pressure inside your eye, which is known as intraocular pressure (IOP). Experts believe this number is a reliable gauge of your glaucoma risk. Early research shows the more active you are, the better your OPP. "We cannot comment on the cause," says study author Paul J. Foster of the University College London Institute of Ophthalmology, "but there is certainly an association between a sedentary lifestyle and factors which increase glaucoma risk."

Secrets to picking eye-saving supplements

Vitamins and herbs may be touted for their eye-helping abilities, but check them out thoroughly before spending your hard-earned money on supplements.

Be smart about vitamins. Although research initially suggested high doses of vitamin C might help prevent cataracts, a recent large study found that neither vitamin E nor vitamin C had any effect. However, newer research shows that vitamin E supplements and B vitamins like riboflavin and thiamin may help slow the progress of cataracts if taken for years. But before taking supplements, make sure you get enough vitamins from your diet, and ask your doctor or pharmacist whether vitamin supplements interfere with medicines you take.

Try a "berry" good idea. Your eyes may benefit from a secret of World War II fighter pilots. They ate bilberry jam regularly to perfect their vision for air missions. Scientists think this European blueberry may help prevent cataracts, especially if you also take other steps to lower your risk. Researchers also suspect bilberry supplements may improve diabetic retinopathy. Just keep in mind that bilberry supplements may have side effects like lowering blood pressure or blood sugar, so talk to your doctor before trying them.

Say no to eyebright. Consider this before you spend money on the herbal supplement eyebright. Professionals say no research supports the use of eyebright for cataracts, and using eyebright as an eye wash puts you at high risk for eye infection. Increases in eye pressure and problems with vision are also possible.

Play the waiting game like a pro

Not everyone needs cataract surgery right away. If you do, your doctor will spot the signs and let you know. Otherwise, you probably don't need it until cataracts interfere with your vision, your ability to drive, or your daily living.

Your doctor may recommend stronger glasses or contact lenses instead of immediate surgery. If that happens, get the most out of your fading vision with these tips.

▸ Use more task lighting, such as lamps that can be placed close to your activity.

▸ Cover shiny tables and other shiny surfaces to reduce glare.

▸ Sit closer to the television.

▸ Assign distinct storage for items that are hard to distinguish. "Containerize" the item in its own box, jar, or tray if needed.

▸ Use different-colored containers for shampoo and conditioner, and use a soap color that shows up clearly against the soap dish.

▸ Put dark-colored drinks and foods in light-colored cups or dishes. Put light-colored edibles in dark dishes.

▸ Ask your pharmacist for prescription labels and drug information sheets in large print.

Get great bargains when surgery can wait

If your vision is fading, use these tricks to get the most quality of life for the least amount of money.

▸ Take advantage of large print books and audio books at your local library.

▸ Take advantage of bargain large print books available from *www.amazon.com*. Go to the book section, and look for a link to the large-print bargain closeout page full of slashed prices.

▸ Help yourself even more with reasonably priced products for low vision. Find page magnifiers, magnifying glasses, large print cookbooks, and much more at Independent Living Aids. Call 800-537-2118 or write to 137 Rano St, Buffalo, NY 14207 to request a free catalog.

Cataract surgery a boon to your brain

Keep an eye on vision changes, and you just may keep your brain sharp as well. People with Alzheimer's disease (AD) can get extra benefits from surgery to remove a cataract.

Researchers identified 38 people suffering from both AD and cataracts. After cataract surgery, all but one person in the study enjoyed improved distance and near vision.

Three months later researchers checked the cognitive abilities of these AD sufferers. For a quarter of the group, the ability to think and interact with the world had improved. Many had less depression, and they slept better. These are the same changes expected in people without dementia after cataract surgery.

Previous research found that people who regularly visit an eye doctor and have their poor vision treated are less likely to develop dementia as they age. All the more reason to take good care of your eyes.

Make surgery more affordable

You may be eligible for free or cheap cataract surgery especially if you can't afford it. If you're uninsured and don't have Medicare or Medicaid, call Mission Cataract USA at 559-797-1629. Leave a message with your name, address, and phone number.

The Knight's Templar Eye Foundation is another source of help for cataract surgery — particularly when government agencies won't fully cover your surgery costs. Check the phone book under Fraternal Organizations, visit *ktef.org*, or write them at 1033 Long Prairie Road, Ste 5, Flower Mound, TX 75022-4230.

Avoid eye surgery dangers

When you agree to cataract surgery, tell your doctor if you've ever taken tamsulosin, other alpha-blocker drugs, or medicines for a urinary tract problem like benign prostatic hyperplasia (BPH.) These medications can cause cataract surgery problems even if you haven't used them lately. Also warn your doctor if you take these medicines:

▸ blood-thinners like warfarin

▸ drugs that affect platelets

▸ latanoprost

▸ steroid eye drops

These drugs can make your surgery more risky, interact with the eye drops you need after surgery, or make your eyes more sensitive to sunlight. Ask your doctor how to avoid these problems, and be sure he knows about any other medicines, herbs, or supplements you take. And don't forget to tell your doctor if you use other eye drops, eye ointments, or eye washes. Taking all your eye products at the same time could be hazardous.

Eye out for a bargain? Spend less on specs

Buying prescription eyeglasses could easily set you back hundreds of dollars. But you can get a brand-new pair for far less. And it doesn't matter where you live because you'll find great deals online. Visit Web sites like *voogueme.com*, *goggles4U.com*, and *zenni optical.com* to browse among hundreds of frames.

Overwhelmed by all the options? Each site offers instructions on how to order and provides tools to narrow your search by shape, material, and size. Some sites even allow you to "try on" frames virtually to see if they suit your face. Prices start at less than $8.

To order, all you'll need is a prescription from your eye doctor. It should include the distance in millimeters between your pupils to ensure a proper focus. And don't pay more by adding a scratch-resistant coating — plastic lenses already have it.

Weigh the pros and cons of multifocal lenses

Cataract surgery usually means new replacement lens implants for your eyes. Standard lens implants can help correct nearsightedness or far-sightedness — but never both. So you'll probably need new reading glasses, regular glasses, or contact lenses after surgery. But if you opt for the newer multifocal lens implants, you may no longer need glasses.

The problem is that Medicare will only reimburse you for the cost of standard lens implants and surgery, so you must pay the cost of the multifocal lenses — usually at least $2,000 out-of-pocket. What's more, these lenses may cause side effects like glare and halos. Talk to your surgeon about the risks, benefits, and prices of these lenses before you decide which ones are right for you.

Colds

Simple, cheap remedies are still the best

Americans suffer a billion colds each year and spend untold time and money trying to cure them. The unpleasant reality is that colds are incurable viral infections. Drugs may ease your symptoms, but the main reason you get better is because your cold has run its course.

Adults average two to four colds a year, usually marked by a stuffy nose, sore throat, and cough. The best treatment is still the time-honored formula of bed rest and fluids. You can search forever for the right medicine — even demand a prescription from the doctor — but in the long run, it will be the simplest and cheapest remedies that do the most good.

No. 1 way to prevent a cold

You don't need special medicines or pills to keep from catching a cold. The best prevention is as simple as washing your hands.

Any one of more than 200 different viruses can give you a cold. You may breathe in airborne germs from coughs or sneezes, but contamination mainly comes from touching something that has a cold virus on it and then touching your eyes, mouth, or nose. When you keep your hands clean, the germs can't get from place to place.

Ordinary soap is all you need. Use warm water, lather up for 15 to 20 seconds, and rinse well. Teach your children and grandchildren to do the same. It's one of the most effective ways to keep from catching or spreading colds and flu.

Waterless, alcohol-based hand cleaners work well when you're not near a sink, but antibacterial soaps offer little protection against viruses. One study suggested that ordinary dishwashing liquid is up to 100 times more effective at killing a virus that causes pneumonia.

Easy way to choose the right remedy

You can spend a lot of time and money at the drugstore and still not get the relief you're looking for. To make it easier, start by checking your symptoms. The exact medicine you need depends on what is bothering you.

For example, if you only have a stuffy nose, just a decongestant will do. For aches and fever, you need a painkiller. Antihistamines relieve itching and sneezing from allergies but don't do much for colds. Cough medicines may include expectorants that thin out mucus when you're congested or suppressants that stop you from coughing.

You can buy each of these ingredients separately and take them according to your symptoms. Or you can buy combination remedies that tackle an assortment of complaints at the same time. The advantage of combinations is they usually cost less overall and they're simpler to take. But make sure you have each of the conditions the ingredients treat so you're not risking side effects for no reason.

When your symptoms last more than two weeks, you may have an allergy, not a cold. Itching, sneezing, and a clear nasal discharge also come from allergies.

Use the chart on the next page to determine which drugs treat the symptoms you have.

Then read the labels before you buy a cold remedy to make sure it contains the drugs you need without unneeded extras. Remember that generic and store brands are less expensive and just as effective as name brands with the same ingredients.

Symptom	Medicine needed	Drug name
stuffy nose	decongestant	pseudoephedrine (Sudafed)
		phenylephrine (Sudafed PE, Neo-synephrine)
coughing	decongestant	See above
	old-style antihistamine	diphenhydramine (Benadryl)
		chlorpheniramine (ChlorTrimeton)
	expectorant	guaifenesin (Robitussin, Mucinex)
	antitussen	dextromethorphan (found in combination remedies)
aches, pain, fever	pain reliever	acetaminophen (Tylenol)

Cut your cold short with natural cures

Time is the only sure cure for a cold. Drugstore medicines can make you more comfortable while you suffer, but a healthy diet, bed rest, and fluids cost less and help just as much. Here are some other natural cures that may help relieve your symptoms.

Boost immunity with echinacea. Consumers spend more than $110 million a year on echinacea to treat or prevent colds. Echinacea supporters say it beefs up your immune system, which fights colds and other infections. Although scientific proof is lacking, it may not hurt to try it — unless you have allergies. Since the echinacea plant is related to daisies and ragweed, it may cause a similar allergic reaction.

Dissolve a zinc lozenge. Take zinc within 24 hours of the sign of a cold and then every two or three waking hours until it goes away, say zinc supporters. It comes as lozenges or a gel and is supposed to strengthen your immunity and shorten the duration of your cold. When buying lozenges, look for zinc gluconate glycine, which is easily released when you suck on the lozenge. Too much zinc can be dangerous though, so don't use it more than three to five days without medical supervision.

> Drinking lots of water can break up thick phlegm just as well as cough medicines with mucus-thinners and expectorant drugs.

Reap the benefits of salt. Home remedies like ordinary table salt are often better than over-the-counter drugs. You can gargle with salt water or use it to wash out your stuffy nose. To soothe your sore throat, gargle several times a day with a quarter to half teaspoon salt in a cup of warm water. The salt relieves the swelling of inflamed throat tissues.

Use a teaspoon of salt in two cups of water to clean out your stuffy nose. Repeat this easy, no-frills method several times a day:

▸ Lean your head over the sink, and pour some of your home-made solution into the palm of your hand.

▸ Inhale the salt-water solution through your nose, one nostril at a time.

▸ Spit out the excess solution, and gently blow your nose.

Sip chicken soup. This folk remedy really works. The warm liquid not only gives you an emotional lift, it soothes your throat and helps clear out your nose. One study concluded chicken soup may contain a number of substances that ease your symptoms. It seems the antioxidants in the vegetables and other ingredients team up to give your body a super anti-inflammatory boost.

Soothe a sore throat with honey. Combine warm liquids and honey to help a sore throat without expensive drugs. Honey eases pain by coating your throat, and its golden goodness is full of compounds that stop bacteria, reduce inflammation, and promote tissue growth. Just the warmth alone from tea, soup, or broth can calm your sore throat and improve circulation.

Foil infections with 2 simple foods

Garlic and yogurt are two foods that act as excellent natural antibiotics and can help you overcome most infections without drugs. Although colds are viral — not bacterial — infections, these foods also boost your overall immune system, which protects you against cold germs along with other infectious invaders.

Garlic has long been a folk remedy for a variety of ills. It is a natural antibiotic that conquers bacteria even some prescription antibiotics can't handle. Plus, it's a flavorful and easy addition to your recipes. A British study found that people taking a daily supplement of allicin — the primary active ingredient in garlic — caught fewer colds and got over them faster than those who took a placebo.

Want even more cold-fighting power? Drink two cups of cranberry juice every day. Experts think the colorful natural compounds in cranberries help fight infection from cold and flu by strengthening your front-line immune cells so you experience fewer symptoms.

Yogurt made from live bacterial cultures is a probiotic. This type of nutrient encourages growth of beneficial bacteria while it strengthens your immune system. A study in Finland found children given milk fortified with live cultures had fewer colds, and workers in Sweden were 55 percent less likely to take sick leave when they took a daily probiotic.

Save money — and your immune system, too

Antibiotics kill bacteria, but they have no effect on the viruses that cause colds and flu. You need an antibiotic only if you suffer complications like strep throat, severe sinusitis, or pneumonia. Don't be one of those people who pressure their doctors into prescribing an antibiotic when an over-the-counter remedy will do. If you get one when you don't need it, you'll not only waste your money, you'll give bacteria a chance to build up an immunity to the drug. Then, when you do need an antibiotic, it may not work.

Beef up your system with a balanced diet

Vitamins — particularly vitamin C — may help prevent and cut short colds under certain circumstances. But you don't need to overload on pills to get the C you need to stop your sniffles. Too many vitamin supplements can throw your system out of balance, not to mention run up your costs.

Most experts recommend foods rich in vitamins A and C, rather than artificial supplements, for help with respiratory infections. It's better to get your vitamins each day from a balanced diet full of fruits and vegetables, light on saturated fats, and free of processed and junk foods. A daily multivitamin may be all the supplement you need.

Experts aren't sure massive doses of vitamin C will stop a cold anyway. You only need 75 mg a day — 90 mg for men — for normal antioxidant protection, and the maximum recommended is 2,000 mg a day. Some advocates suggest taking up to 4,000 mg for a cold, but too much vitamin C can lead to side effects like bloating and diarrhea. It may also make you absorb too much iron, lead to kidney stones, or erode the enamel on your teeth. Plus, vitamin C is water soluble, and if you take in more than you need, your body will simply flush it away.

A little extra vitamin E may be helpful, though. A Tufts University study found elderly nursing home residents who took 200 IU of vitamin E a day had fewer colds. The usual recommended daily intake is 33 IU.

Feeling crummy? Breathe easier with probiotics

What if you could have an army of billions fighting your next upper respiratory infection (URI)? You can — with probiotics, shows a study published in the *British Journal of Nutrition*.

The bacteria *Lactobacillus rhamnosus* (LGG) and *Bifidobacterium animalis* (BB-12) shortened the duration of URIs by two days and lowered the severity of infections by 34 percent. The supplements used in the study were powders that could form bacteria by the billions. Scientists believe these beneficial bugs work by lowering the inflammation associated with URIs.

Want to give these a try? You can find *Lactobacillus rhamnosus* (LGG) in products like yogurt drinks all over the world, but in the U.S., it's primarily in supplements. Read labels carefully.

And *Bifidobacterium animalis* (BB-12) is found in both yogurts and supplements. Look for the words *B. animalis*, *B. lactis*, or *B. regularis* on labels.

Dollars&Sense
Free or low-cost Rx drugs at any age

Believe it or not, you could qualify for free medication even if you're under age 65. In fact, some people with insurance or Medicare Part D still get help with their drug costs. Discover the variety of options that could ease the hardship of paying for your prescription drugs.

Get wise to Patient Assistance Programs. Drug companies offer Patient Assistance Programs (PAPs) to help people living on low incomes get free medication. You're most likely to qualify if you are ineligible for other assistance programs.

Plan to apply separately for each medication you take and be ready to provide proof-of-income documents. Your doctor or another health professional must also fill out forms on your behalf, so be prepared. And don't hesitate to fill prescriptions you'll use soon. It could take several weeks to find out if you qualify.

You may have heard you won't qualify for assistance if you enroll in Medicare Part D. But some programs have declared Part D participants eligible again. Regardless of whether you're enrolled in Part D or not, contact these organizations to find programs you might qualify for.

▸ **Partnership for Prescription Assistance (PPA).** Visit *medicineassistancetool.org*. You'll find more than 180 drug company PAPs and dozens of other programs for free or low-cost drugs.

▸ **RxAssist.org.** Visit *www.rxassist.org*. The Web site includes application forms for some programs, but you must register for a free account to use the site.

▸ **NeedyMeds.com.** Visit *www.needymeds.org* or call 800-503-6897. You'll find drug company PAPs plus government programs, discount drug cards, and generic drug assistance.

▸ **BenefitsCheckUp.** Visit *www.benefitscheckup.org* if you're 55 or older. Learn which programs you qualify for if you don't have Medicare Part D, or if you have Part D, check whether you're eligible for additional savings from the "Extra Help" program.

▸ **Together Rx Access.** Apply for the Together Rx Access drug discount card for up to 40 percent off medications from 10 big-name drug companies. To qualify you must meet income requirements, be ineligible for Medicare, and have no pre-scription drug coverage. Visit *www.togetherrxaccess.com.*

Slash insurance copays. If you have insurance, help is available for steep copayments that cause financial hardship.

▸ **Patient Services, Inc.** Get up to two years of copay assis-tance for selected illnesses and conditions. Call 800-366-7741 or visit *patientservicesinc.org/* for more information.

▸ **Patient Advocate Foundation Co-Pay Relief.** Call 866-512-3861 or visit *www.copays.org* to find out the medical and financial requirements for this program. You can qualify even if you have Medicare Part D.

Sign up for discount programs. Grocery stores and drug-stores are always trying to get more customers in the door. Some have even started offering pharmacy discounts. If you're a savvy shopper, these loyalty programs can help you save hundreds on your meds.

You might have to pay a small annual membership fee, but in return you'll get the lowest prices on medications.

Make sure you know exactly what the programs offer before you sign up. And check to see if they'll actually help you save money. The program may not offer discounts on every medica-tion, or you might not be able to use them if you have Medicare Part D.

Constipation

Ease the discomfort for less

"More than $700 million" may sound like the budget for a blockbuster movie, but that's how much Americans spend on over-the-counter laxatives every year. What's more, several million people say they feel constipated most of the time.

Constipation happens when the muscles in your colon, or large intestine, move waste along too slowly. As a result, your colon withdraws too much water from the waste, leaving you with dry, hard stool and constipation.

If your constipation doesn't improve after a week, see your doctor. Constipation can be a symptom of many serious conditions. But if your doctor says disease isn't the cause of your problem, there are simple, inexpensive ways to find relief.

Surprising cause of irregularity

Lack of fiber contributes to constipation, but it isn't the only cause. Over-the-counter cold, flu, or allergy medicines could also be making you constipated, warns drug watchdog, worstpills.org. Check the labels on your drugs. Limit or avoid the ones that contain chlorpheniramine, clemastine, or brompheniramine. What's more, some antacids can lead to constipation, too. Bypass the ones that contain aluminum hydroxide, magnesium hydroxide, or

calcium carbonate. Iron and calcium supplements are also culprits. Ask your doctor or pharmacist to suggest good substitutes.

And don't forget to check your prescription medicines. Drugs
like these can also cause constipation or make it worse.

- sedatives and antidepressants
- diuretics
- cough syrups with codeine
- painkillers that contain narcotics
- lovastatin

Talk to your doctor or pharmacist. Ask whether medicines you
take might make you constipated and what you should do about it.
You might be able to switch to another medicine or take a lower dose.
Getting back to normal could be just that easy. Just remember —
never stop taking a drug your doctor prescribed without his approval.

Thrifty ways to get more fiber

Fiber doesn't have to carry a big price tag, and these tips can help
you prove it.

- Wash fruits and veggies and eat the skin, along with the delicious interior. It won't cost you one penny extra.

- Add canned or dry beans to soups and stews. Beans and other
legumes are inexpensive and a great source of fiber. To avoid gas,
start with small amounts and gradually add more — or soak dried
beans, discard the water, and rinse the beans before cooking.

- Compare cereal prices. Cereals with dried fruit already added
may cost more than tossing your own sliced or dried fruit into
plain cereal.

- Trade low-fiber foods, like candies, puddings, cakes, and pas-
tries, for fresh fruits, like apples and figs, and crisp, raw veggies.

Don't be surprised if the produce costs less. Store-bought goodies can be pricey.

Eating whole grains, fruits, vegetables, and legumes is the best — and cheapest — way to increase your fiber intake. These foods offer vital nutrients and delicious taste that laxatives don't have, and you'll avoid dangerous side effects, too.

Get tough with fiber

Fiber comes in two varieties — insoluble and soluble. Each has its own set of benefits, but both can help keep your digestive tract healthy and move waste through your colon like an expess subway train.

▸ Insoluble fiber adds bulk and speeds food through your digestive system. It also softens stool so it's easy to pass. Foods high in insoluble fiber include whole grains, wheat bran, fruits, veggies, legumes, brown rice, and popcorn.

▸ Soluble fiber dissolves easily in water. It makes food gummy or gel-like, helping it move along faster. It also helps soak up extra cholesterol and keep your blood sugar under control. You can get it from fruits, veggies, seeds, rye, oats, barley, rice bran, peas, and beans.

4 ways to beat constipation — for free

If you've relied on laxatives in the past, now is the time to try natural ways to keep your digestive tract on a regular schedule.

▸ Take a walk every day. A mild workout like this stimulates your bowels naturally.

▸ Schedule a visit to the bathroom at the same time every day, perhaps after a meal or upon waking. Pick an idle part of the day so you won't try to rush or strain. But if you need to go at another time, don't wait.

▸ Massage your abdominal area in a clockwise motion. Some natural healers believe this helps relieve constipation.

▸ Try sitting quietly for 15 to 20 minutes each day, focusing on deep, even breathing. Other simple relaxation techniques may work well, too.

Gut check: Be proactive with probiotics

Ever wonder why so many places — from gas stations to fast-food chains — keep a stock of yogurt cups, yogurt bars, and yogurt parfaits? Maybe it's because this creamy, delicious treat serves up health benefits by the billions — billions of probiotics, that is. As a form of good bacteria, they help you digest food, fight off illness, and maintain a healthy gut. Perhaps even keep you regular, since studies show probiotics make your stools softer, speed up your stool's travel time, and help you go more often.

While yogurt is a tasty way to get probiotics, you can also buy probiotic tablets, capsules, and softgels. Researchers identified the *Bifidobacterium lactis* strain as delivering the most constipation relief when they examined multiple studies. So look for that on the label.

> Adding too much fiber too fast can lead to gas and other uncomfortable symptoms that often make people avoid fiber altogether. Build up your intake slowly for long-term success.

In addition, a study out of Italy had people with chronic constipation take a tablet containing 100 million cells of the strain *Lactobacillus reuteri* twice a day, 30 minutes after eating. After four weeks, they reported going more often per week with softer stools.

Even people with constipation caused by irritable bowel syndrome (IBS) may benefit from taking probiotics or eating yogurt. Experts now believe chronic constipation and IBS may belong to the same family of medical conditions.

Watch out for whole grain imposters

When you read the ingredient list for a product, don't be fooled by terms like "100% wheat," "enriched flour," "multigrain," "wheat flour," "degerminated cornmeal," or "stone ground." These don't guarantee that a product is "whole grain." Instead, check for terms like whole oats, whole wheat, oatmeal, whole rye, cracked wheat, whole grain corn, pearl barley, brown rice, or graham flour.

3 everyday foods that cure constipation

Is constipation a constant in your daily life? Have you tried laxatives, fiber supplements, and folk remedies with no relief? Good news — you can stop searching. Eating these three foods every day is a proven way to get regular.

Olive, not mineral, oil for less straining. Olive oil relieves constipation just as well as mineral oil. Plus, it's full of nutrients and healthy fats that fight inflammation. In one study, constipated people began taking about one teaspoon of either olive oil or mineral oil every day. After four weeks, roughly six out of 10 people were no longer constipated. Surprisingly, the olive oil group had the highest "cured" rate.

Both oils have the same effect — lubricating and softening stool to help it move through your intestines. But unlike olive oil, mineral oil has no nutritional value. Even worse, it's made from petroleum. Olive oil, especially the extra virgin type, is packed with nutrients

Add more fiber, juiciness, and taste appeal to your sandwiches. Spruce them up with sliced green or red sweet peppers, lettuce, sliced carrots, spinach leaves, cucumbers, or tomato.

and health benefits. People in this study saw relief with as little as one teaspoon of oil, but others who tried it on their own used two tablespoons safely and with success.

Kiwi can help you go. This little wonder fruit fits the bill for people suffering from constipation. Kiwi fiber can hold lots of water, which helps soften and bulk up stool so it's easier to pass. But that's just for starters. Kiwis also contain an enzyme that stimulates your colon, helping stool move through your bowels faster. The time it takes stool to move through your colon directly affects how often you have bowel movements. Slower movement equals fewer bowel movements and potentially more constipation.

Research suggests that eating two kiwis each day can treat both regular constipation and constipation linked to irritable bowel syndrome (IBS).

▸ After eating two kiwis a day for four weeks, half of people with constipation were having more bowel movements and needed laxatives less often.

▸ Eating two kiwis a day in another study began to ease IBS-related constipation after just one week. People had bowel movements more often, and stool passed through their colons faster.

The best thing about this fruit? It's natural. Unlike laxatives, eating a couple of kiwis doesn't seem to cause any side effects, unless you are allergic to them. The longer you eat them, the more they seem to improve constipation.

Bread swap can get you moving again. Rethink your daily bread. Making your sandwiches out of whole-grain rye, not white wheat bread, could relieve constipation. Rye contains a type of fiber called arabinoxylan that gets fermented by bacteria in your colon.

That fermentation produces compounds that cause your colon to contract, moving stool along faster and relieving constipation.

Fifty-one people with constipation tested the effects of swapping rye bread for white wheat in their diets. For three weeks, they either:

▸ ate six slices of whole-grain rye each day, for a total of 30 grams of fiber.

▸ ate eight slices of low-fiber white wheat bread, for 8.6 grams of fiber.

▸ or took laxatives.

The rye won, hands down, easing constipation even more than laxatives.

Supplement warning you should not ignore

Taking fiber supplements, including the herb psyllium, could interfere with the absorption of medications you take and minerals you need. Fiber sweeps them through your digestive system without giving them time to get fully absorbed.

• Medications — If you take drugs for your heart, cholesterol, or diabetes, experts suggest taking fiber supplements two to three hours before or after you take your medications. These include popular prescriptions like Crestor, Plavix, and Lipitor.

• Minerals — Your body needs iron, zinc, calcium, and magnesium for good health. But eating too much fiber can bind with these minerals and flush them out of your body before you can absorb them. Stick to eating the recommended daily allowance — 25 grams a day for women and 38 grams a day for men — and fiber shouldn't be a problem.

Sweet solution for stubborn constipation

The Greeks have known it for years, but now the secret is out. Fast relief from constipation could be hiding in your kitchen cupboard. Old-fashioned honey may be all you need to get your bowels moving.

Honey contains three types of sugar — glucose, fructose, and sucrose. Natural honeys pack more fructose than glucose. Experts think that imbalance can help loosen stool.

In most people, the small intestine can't completely absorb fructose. The result is a little like what happens when people who are lactose-intolerant drink milk. The excess fructose causes the small intestine to hold more water and sends food through the digestive tract faster.

A single dose should do the trick. Start by mixing one-and-a-half tablespoons of honey in a glass of water, the usual dose for treating constipation in Greece. This small amount had a laxative effect in one study. Wait at least 10 hours. If it hasn't helped, you can increase the dose to three tablespoons.

Drink more water and other liquids as you boost the fiber in your diet. Increasing your fiber intake without adding extra fluids can make your constipation worse.

Honey may not work for everyone, but it could help some. Out of 20 people, three responded to the smaller dose, while six responded to the larger dose. You may want to avoid this home remedy if you have irritable bowel syndrome, though. The extra fructose could aggravate your digestive tract.

Depression

Self-help strategies and money-saving tips

Feeling a little down in the dumps is one thing. Depression is quite another. When you suffer from depression, you may feel overwhelming sadness, lose interest in things you once enjoyed, have trouble sleeping, or experience changes in appetite or weight. You might also have trouble concentrating or making decisions; feel guilty, worthless, or hopeless; and often think of death or suicide.

The cause of depression remains unknown, but chemical imbalances in the brain, genetic factors, B-vitamin deficiencies, certain medications, and illness are all possible causes.

Depression is a serious medical condition. You can't just "snap out of it." You need professional help. The most common treatment options include medication, therapy, or a combination of the two. But you can also take some steps to help yourself. Read on to discover these self-help strategies and alternatives to prescription pills.

Top tips for beating the blues

When you're feeling blue, you can perk yourself up with these simple strategies.

Exercise your cares away. Many studies have found that moderate to strenuous exercise can help brighten your mood while it strengthens your body. A recent study found exercise to be as effective as medication or therapy for mild to moderate depression. People in the study, who exercised on a treadmill or on a stationary bicycle three to five times a week, reduced their depression symptoms by nearly 50 percent after 12 weeks. The key is to exercise at a moderate intensity at least 30 minutes a day most days of the week. Choose an activity you particularly enjoy so you'll be more likely to stick with it.

Surround yourself with music. You always knew it was true, and now science proves it. Music can cheer you up. Just by listening to music, people suffering from chronic pain reduced their depression up to 25 percent. Music works to calm your nerves whether you listen to classical or jazz or take part in making it. Researchers in the field of music therapy say that playing a specially designed music-making computer program, playing an instrument, or just singing along with others reduces stress.

Pamper yourself with massage. Don't think of a massage as overindulgence — think of it as an investment in your good health. Research has shown that various forms of massage, from the relaxing Swedish massage to the invigorating aromatherapy massage, can help lower blood pressure as well as your heart rate. On top of that, certain essential oils used in aromatherapy massage may help relieve depression. Find a qualified massage therapist through the locator service of the American Massage Therapy Association by calling toll free 877–905–2700 or going online at *www.amtamassage.org*.

Herbal remedy blasts the blahs

Mild depression should not put a major dent in your wallet. Instead of costly prescription drugs, try a proven natural remedy. Studies show that St. John's wort, an over-the-counter herbal supplement,

works as well as standard antidepressants with fewer side effects
— at a fraction of the cost.

A one-month supply of St.
John's wort costs around $12.
The standard dosage is 900 milligrams a day. You can take two
450-mg doses or three 300-mg
doses. Look for standardized
formulations. Otherwise, you're
not sure what you're getting.

If neither drugs nor therapy
relieve your depression,
consider an implanted pace-
maker-like device that sends
electrical pulses to your
brain. The technique, called
vagus nerve stimulation, may
have long-lasting effects.

Remember, St. John's wort should only be used as a short-term
treatment for mild depression. Major depression usually requires
prescription drugs.

Do not take St. John's wort if you're already taking a prescription
antidepressant. A dangerous reaction called serotonin syndrome
could result. St. John's wort may also interact with other drugs, so
it's important to let your doctor know you are taking it.

Lighten your load with light therapy

Just as there is a baseball season or hurricane season, some people
experience a depression season. For people with seasonal affective
disorder (SAD), the winter months and their lack of sunlight can
bring on depression. Researchers think changes in the levels of certain brain chemicals might be responsible.

Because darkness seems to trigger SAD, it makes sense that light
could help cure it. Although not much solid research exists, the few
well-designed studies do support this theory. In fact, light therapy
seems to help people with regular depression as well as those with
SAD. Light therapy may even work as well as some antidepressants.

The key is the bright artificial light, measured in units called lux and delivered through a special light box. Typical therapy is at 10,000 lux and involves sessions lasting from 30 minutes to two hours a day. Just sitting near the light box does the trick. You could read, listen to music, or watch TV. Usually, early morning is the best time for light therapy.

You can buy 10,000-lux light boxes on the Internet or in some drugstores or hardware stores. Prices range from $200 to $500. Some health insurance companies will cover the cost.

Light therapy comes with some safety concerns. Possible side effects include headache, eyestrain, nausea, and agitation. What's more, some products are unsafe or ineffective. Make sure you talk to your doctor before trying light therapy on your own.

3 foods to improve your state of mind

When you feel depressed, maybe you turn to food. Sweets, like ice cream, cookies, and chocolate, may seem like just what the doctor ordered, but they'll actually leave you feeling worse a short time later. Try these foods to help lift your spirits.

▸ **Fish.** Low fish consumption has been linked to depression. A recent Finnish study found that women who rarely ate fish were more than twice as likely to develop depression as those who regularly ate fish. The omega-3 fatty acids found in fish work wonders for your brain. Eating more cold-water fish, like salmon, sardines, and herring, or taking fish oil capsules can give you the omega-3 you need.

▸ **Saffron.** A small Iranian study found this staple of traditional Persian medicine to be effective in treating mild depression. The study used saffron capsules, but you can try adding some of this popular Middle Eastern spice to your dishes. It's expensive, however. An ounce of saffron costs over $100.

- **Fortified breads and cereals.** Low levels of folate, a B vitamin, have also been linked to depression. Besides fortified breads and cereals, you can find folate in legumes, seeds, and dark green leafy vegetables. Folic acid supplements are also available.

The healing power of tea time

The soothing rhythm of preparing tea may do wonders for your mental state. But the biggest benefit may be in the tea itself. Drinking 1 or more cups a day is an easy way to get nutrients that work together to fight depression.

Researchers believe the combination of chemicals in tea, rather than one in particular, may give tea its anti-depression powers. Each makes a small change that leads to an overall difference in your mood.

Multifunctional tea takes down depression. Like grapes, tea impacts the major paths scientists believe control depression. For instance, your HPA axis manages your fight-or-flight response. If stress causes it to operate continuously, referred to as HPA axis hyperactivity, it can overwhelm you and lead to symptoms of depression. But the polyphenols in tea may help normalize its activity.

> More women than men experience depression. In fact, depression strikes up to 25 percent of women at some point in their lives.

Tea has also been shown to lower inflammation, help rebalance neurotransmitters like serotonin and dopamine, and fight oxidation that damages neurons — all of which can lead to depression.

Keep the cups flowing for best results. Don't worry about what kind of tea you're drinking for now. Scientists aren't sure which type is the best, and since each tea has its own beneficial qualities, your best bet may actually be to drink multiple types regularly.

What matters more is how much you drink. Studies have found that a higher consumption of tea is linked with lower risk of depression.

- In an analysis of 11 studies, researchers found that for every 3 cups of tea you drink in a day there is an associated 37 percent decrease in risk of depression.

- Examination of a Korean survey of health and nutrition found that those who drank more than 3 cups of green tea in a week had 21 percent lower rates of depression.

Aging populations especially seem to benefit from tea's depression-reducing effects. However, it works best in mild to moderate cases and may not make a significant dent in severe depression.

One yummy snack for a happier you

Move over double chocolate ice cream. There's a new comfort food in town, and it's actually good for you.

Long thought of as a way to build better bones and keep trim, yogurt's benefits may extend to your mood. Who would have thought a simple trip to the dairy aisle could pep up your step?

High-fat yogurt keeps you in high spirits. A recent study from Spain says eating whole-fat yogurt may help ward off depression. Women who ate a half cup of the yogurt at least seven times a week were less likely to develop depression than those who ate the same amount less than once a week. Low-fat yogurt didn't have the same effect.

Scientists don't know what causes depression, but they do say it may be linked to low-grade inflammation and a lack of folate in the diet. That's where whole-fat yogurt steps in. It contains more folate than the fat-free variety. And experts think healthy fats fight inflammation.

More fat doesn't mean more calories. High-fat yogurt won't pack on the pounds. In fact, an 8-ounce container of plain, whole-milk yogurt contains just 149 calories. Oddly enough, the same amount of low-fat yogurt has 154 calories. Pull out your reading glasses, scan the nutrition label, and you'll find the reason why. The low-fat version has almost 6 more grams of sugar than the high-fat kind.

Amazing way to relieve depression

Try an easy, five-minute, four-step method that lowers blood pressure, relieves depression, and improves the immune system of cancer patients — without drugs or pills of any kind. It's called progressive muscle relaxation, and here's how to do it.

▸ Find a quiet, comfortable place to sit.

▸ Start by taking a few slow, deep breaths.

▸ Close your eyes and gradually relax the muscles of your body, one group at a time. Begin by clenching the muscles of your toes while you count to 10, then relax them for a count of 10.

▸ Tense and relax your leg muscles, then move on through the other muscle groups in your entire body. By the time you get to your head, you should feel more calm.

Bacteria boost your brain. Fermentation, which gives yogurt that classic tangy flavor, is caused by friendly bacteria. These good guys may also put you in a good mood. That's because certain strains of *lactobacillus* help keep your brain in balance, studies say.

India's gold can brighten your mood

Caught with your hand in the cookie jar a little too often? Napping all afternoon instead of visiting friends? Forgot where you left your car keys again?

Overeating, oversleeping, and forgetfulness are just a few of the many signs of depression. This all-too-common illness can make you feel as if the whole world has lost its color, its vibrant hues turned to gray. A sprinkle of bright orange turmeric — also known as India's gold — may be just what you need to beat the blues.

Brighten your world with a simple kitchen spice. People with depression often suffer from chronic inflammation that lowers the amount of the brain chemicals dopamine and serotonin. These feel-good neurotransmitters are in charge of brain functions like mood and motivation. So if you're cheerfully cleaning out that closet you've been wanting to tackle, you can bet your levels are high. Curcumin provides a natural way to boost dopamine and serotonin so you can enjoy those positive feelings more often.

Experts have learned when you're depressed, your body also undergoes more oxidative stress. That means harmful molecules called free radicals are flooding your system, sending all the major organs in your body — including your brain — into a tailspin. Turmeric's power player, curcumin, is a natural antioxidant that can fend off those destructive free radicals and help prevent a downward spiral.

How to ditch the moody blues. In one Chinese study, scientists tested curcumin on more than 100 men suffering with depression. Volunteers were asked to take two capsules containing 1,000 milligrams (mg) of either curcumin or soybean powder every day. After six weeks, a standard depression questionnaire showed the curcumin group's symptoms improved significantly compared to the soy group.

Another study followed more than 50 people with major depressive disorder who received either 500 mg of curcumin twice each day or a placebo for eight weeks. Again, people taking curcumin felt significantly better than those on the placebo, especially after four to eight weeks.

Comfort creatures — why your pet is good for you

No question, a playful pooch can be a joy and a comfort, especially if you're feeling down or anxious. Experts say just turn to that little tail-wagger for some "bone"-a fide therapy.

Studies show interacting with a pet, particularly dogs, means less anxiety, depression, loneliness, and boredom. In addition, spending time with your beloved animals may lower your heart rate and blood pressure.

Even if you don't own a pet, happy time can be just around the corner. Visit an animal shelter or volunteer to walk your neighbor's dog.

Dollars&Sense
Watch out for Medicare Rx scams

Every year you get a golden opportunity to enroll in a Medicare prescription drug plan that saves you money. But make sure you don't end up losing money by giving your business to an illegal provider. Here's what you need to know.

Medicare has teamed up with private companies to offer Part D prescription drug coverage to everyone eligible for Medicare. Although the plans conform to Medicare's standards, their features, list of drugs covered, and their costs can vary widely. So you need information from the plans to make the best choice.

That's where the scam artists come in. They pose as government officials or representatives for Part D plans. They may call, e-mail, or even visit your home to sell fake plans or a new Medicare card. They may say they need payment for an enrollment fee or some other cost, but they really want your bank account number, credit card number, or other personal information.

Avoid the scams. If someone contacts you about a Medicare prescription plan, remember these points.

▸ You can only sign up for a Part D plan during the October 15 to December 7 enrollment period. Be suspicious of anyone who contacts you at other times of the year.

▸ Legitimate Medicare providers should not ask for your bank account number or for payment over the phone or Internet. They should bill you or mail you an offer for automatic withdrawal.

▸ Part D plans have no enrollment fee.

▸ Medicare plan providers cannot use unsolicited e-mails or uninvited door-to-door sales calls.

▸ Providers should be willing to mail you information about their plan — and wait for you to review it — before you enroll in a plan.

▸ Don't enroll in a plan during the first phone call. Instead, ask for the company's name and phone number. Then call 800-633-4227 to check whether the caller's company is a legitimate Medicare plan provider.

Ask money-saving questions. Even if the caller turns out to be legitimate, don't enroll in any plan until you get answers to questions like these.

▸ Would this plan cover my current medications? If it doesn't, it's not much use to you. At the very least, you need one that covers your most expensive drugs.

▸ Can I use my regular pharmacy? Others may not charge the same prices.

▸ What will my medications cost per month? What co-pays, deductibles, and premiums can I expect?

▸ When will the plan stop paying for my drugs? Part D plans have a point at which they will no longer cover your drug costs until you pay an additional amount. Find out whether the plan will provide any benefits within this coverage gap.

These questions are a good start, but you need more information to make a money-saving decision. For example, some people who have prescription drug coverage will save money by sticking with it instead of enrolling in Part D. Yet others should enroll in Part D to avoid financial penalties.

Medicare personnel can help you figure out what to do. They can also provide publications to help you pick a plan. Call 800-633-4227 or visit *www.medicare.gov* for more information.

Diabetes

Manage blood sugar and minimize cost

Almost 34 million Americans have diabetes, and many don't know it. While the death rates from heart disease and cancer have been dropping, the death rate for diabetes has been going up.

Although diabetes can be deadly, there are plenty of things you can do to keep it under control. Some are simple, like getting more exercise and watching what you eat. Others involve checking your blood sugar and asking your doctor about new diabetes drugs. Either way, dealing with diabetes requires lifestyle changes to help you avoid severe complications, like heart disease, kidney failure, blindness, and amputations.

'Miracle cure' in your medicine cabinet

New research has uncovered some amazing possibilities for aspirin. In fact, the American Diabetes Association suggests that people with diabetes take an aspirin a day to cut their risk of heart disease. Aspirin in small, regular doses helps prevent blood clots from forming, which reduces your risk of heart attack and stroke. For people with diabetes, aspirin also helps by warding off diabetic retinopathy, which can result in blindness.

But the benefits of aspirin don't end there. Recent studies on overweight mice showed that aspirin in extremely high doses reversed some signs of type 2 diabetes and reduced low-grade inflammation, which is linked to insulin resistance.

Insulin is a hormone that turns blood sugar into energy. When your body resists insulin, sugar builds up in your blood. Dangerously high levels of blood sugar can damage your heart, blood vessels, kidneys, and eyes.

The high doses of aspirin used in the study effectively reversed diabetes in the mice. Researchers are now investigating how this high-dose aspirin therapy might work on people. Unfortunately, regular aspirin use can cause major bleeding and harm your liver and kidneys.

> About 40 to 50 percent of people with diabetes don't take their medicine correctly. Follow instructions on the package carefully. If there's anything you don't understand, call your doctor or pharmacist.

For now, ask your doctor if you should try daily, low-dose aspirin therapy to reduce your risk of heart attack and stroke. Even though researchers have known for a long time about the benefits of aspirin therapy for diabetics, only about 12 percent of people with diabetes take aspirin regularly.

2 great reasons to go for a walk

Doctors often turn to drugs to treat diabetes. Unfortunately, a common side effect of many popular diabetes meds is weight gain, which can make your symptoms worse. The good news? Simply taking a walk can help you keep your appetite down and your blood sugar in check.

Get moving to control cravings. Aerobic exercises like walking and jogging seem to suppress appetite, in general, by boosting your blood levels of brain-derived neurotrophic factor (BDNF). This protein helps keep nerve cells healthy, but it may also suppress appetite. One study found that exercising upped BDNF levels in overweight and obese people. The higher their BDNF, the more weight they lost and the fewer calories they ate.

Aerobic exercise also stimulates the appetite-suppressing hormone peptide YY and squashes the appetite-boosting hormone ghrelin. So go for a walk after dinner to feel less hungry and stimulate gradual weight loss.

Pick up the pace for better blood sugar. Are you discouraged by the thought of completely changing your lifestyle to avoid diabetes? Then do this one thing. Go out for a fast walk.

People who took moderately intense walks of 11 to 14 miles per week — that's less than two miles a day — lowered their blood sugar levels almost as effectively as people who combined three lifestyle changes — diet, exercise, and weight loss.

Want to count steps instead of miles? Some experts suggest a goal of 10,000 steps a day. Why not take the stairs or park your car

Can't-miss tips for workout safety

Exercising when you have diabetes means taking a few extra precautions.

▸ Wear a medical ID bracelet or other identification that lets people know you have diabetes. Include your name, address, and phone number; your doctor's information; and a list of your medications and doses.

▸ Carry a blood glucose monitor with you if you plan an extra-long workout.

▸ Take glucose tablets or hard candy with you in case of low blood sugar.

at the far end of a parking lot. To make it easier to track your progress, get a fitness watch or app for your smartphone. Just make sure your steps are fast ones.

Ancient herb controls sugar, boosts energy

Feeling tired all the time? The herb ginseng, used in traditional Chinese medicine, not only lowers blood sugar in type 2 diabetics, it also raises energy levels.

Sometimes known as the "king herb," ginseng has long been trusted as a treatment for diabetes and other ailments. Ancient Chinese healers have used the plant for 2,000 years. For decades, its main active ingredients, ginsenosides, have been isolated from the ginseng root to treat the high blood sugar of diabetes. Ginsenosides from both the American ginseng and the Asian ginseng plant can help balance blood sugar levels and increase the amount of insulin in the blood. Repeated, high-quality research has tested the effects in numerous studies.

But what about the rest of the ginseng plant? Now scientists are using ginseng berries, which contain more of the compound ginsenoside Re — one type of ginsenoside — to see how diabetic symptoms can be reduced. Researchers at the University of Chicago tested ginseng berry extract on overweight mice with type 2 diabetes to see how blood sugar and weight were affected.

Australian researchers found drinking at least 8 ounces of clarified, or filtered, tomato juice a day lowered the risk for atherosclerosis, heart attack, and stroke in type 2 diabetics.

Mice who received the extract every day showed improved blood sugar levels. They also had better scores on a glucose-tolerance test, which shows how fast the mice removed excess blood sugar from their blood. In addition, the mice lost weight — about 10 percent of their body weight in 12 days — because they ate less and were more active. When the ginseng berry injections stopped, the mice regained the weight. A control group of nondiabetic, normal-weight mice didn't show any of these changes.

Other studies have shown similar effects from ginseng berry extract, making it a great candidate to treat diabetes. The leaf of the ginseng plant, which contains even more ginsenosides of different types than the root or berry, has also shown promise for controlling blood sugar. More research needs to be done, however, to prove the success of ginseng leaf for people with diabetes.

Get control of your diabetes with help from fiber

A 12-week study of people with type 2 diabetes found that those who ate a high-fiber diet had greater reductions in their average fasting glucose levels than a control group on a standard diet. They also lost more weight.

The researchers say the high-fiber diet promoted the growth of gut bacteria that produced short-chain fatty acids. The acids made the intestinal tracts of the fiber-eating participants less hospitable to harmful bacteria. The result? The amount of bad bacteria in their guts dropped. The acids also led to increases in insulin production and better glucose control, the scientists say.

Avoid this dangerous intersection between gum disease and diabetes

Inflammation is a key part of gum disease and diabetes. And scientists now believe these two conditions may actually fuel one another.

Call on this humble spice to lower your blood sugar

Would you believe that cinnamon oils can help heal wounds? Even better, studies have shown this spice can lower your cholesterol and blood pressure, fight inflammation and cancer, and fend off fatigue and food poisoning. It's even on the cutting edge of Alzheimer's prevention.

But the best part? Sprinkling a bit more of this sweet spice on your meals may help you fight back against diabetes.

In a recent meta-analysis, researchers examined multiple studies and found cinnamon can lower your fasting blood sugar and even improve your insulin resistance. But other research findings have been mixed.

If you want to give it a try, talk to your doctor about a safe amount to take. Some studies have used up to 6 grams of cinnamon a day, which is about 2 1/3 teaspoons. If you have liver problems, eating too much cinnamon could make them worse. So be smart and take your doctor's advice.

How? The bacteria that causes gum disease can migrate into your bloodstream. Naturally your body will put up a fight. That's good, but compounds produced by your immune reaction may raise your blood sugar. So if you have an ongoing problem like gum disease, then you could be setting yourself up with higher blood sugar levels over the long term. And that can lead to type 2 diabetes.

The reverse also seems to be true. People with unchecked diabetes run a higher risk of inflammation and gum disease. One possible reason? Diabetes can damage the blood vessels that supply nutrients to your gums. That can make it harder to fight infection.

So what should you do? Keep your gums healthy by brushing gently twice a day, and get regular checkups and cleanings.

Action plan for low blood sugar

If you take insulin for diabetes, you may be plagued by episodes of hypoglycemia, or low blood sugar. Doctors say to treat these incidents by eating about 15 grams of a fast-acting carbohydrate, like glucose. Special tablets and gels contain pure glucose, but candy with sucrose, or table sugar, also works — just not as fast. Candy bars and other treats with chocolate contain lots of fat, which slows digestion and the absorption of sugar. They should be your last choice.

Women with diabetes are at higher risk for hip fractures. A long-term study shows the risk is doubled for women with type 2 diabetes and six times higher with type 1 diabetes.

You should not eat diabetic snack bars or meal bars, like Extend Nutrition bars or NiteBite, if you have an episode of low blood sugar. These bars are made to prevent low blood sugar, and they act too slowly.

Smart advice for buying a glucose monitor

People with diabetes must keep a close eye on their blood sugar levels. You may have to check your glucose a dozen or more times each day. Using an up-to-date glucose monitor that's made for home use can really help keep your blood sugar under control. Dozens of styles are available for a wide range of prices. Here are some features to consider before you buy.

Cost. Before you make a purchase, check with your insurance company to see what products are covered. Machines can range from less than $100 to more than $700 if you have to foot the bill. Also, remember that the cost of test strips, which you need each time you test and are specific to each monitor, will probably be higher than the cost of the machine over time. You'll want to factor that difference into your choice.

Features you need. Some monitors made for sight-impaired people give verbal directions for each step in the testing process and an audio output of the results. Sounds handy, but these monitors are the most expensive.

Ease of use. All of the new monitors are small, light, and portable, with some weighing just a few ounces. Try to "test drive" a few models to see how comfortable they feel in your hand and whether the screen is easy to read. Other features to consider include how much blood is needed and how long you must wait for results.

Accuracy. All meters on the market are quite accurate if you use them correctly. Be sure to check the readings at least once a month to calibrate your monitor. Some monitors calibrate themselves, while others require extra steps.

Record-keeping. Many monitors store test results for days or weeks at a time, but you may want even more information. Data-management systems can help you keep track of information such as glucose reading, date, time, food eaten, exercise levels — everything you and your doctor need to know to keep your blood sugar under control.

Alternate testing sites. Some monitors let you test blood that is drawn from sites other than your fingertips, making for less-painful testing. Ask your doctor if it's right for you.

Once you've bought a glucose monitor, read the directions and use it carefully. The Food and Drug Administration (FDA) has had reports of people accidentally changing the units of measurement on their monitors, which can cause the reading to appear to be 18 times higher or lower than it really is. So be careful when you change the time or date on your monitor, and check the settings if you accidentally drop it.

Hit the road with fewer hassles

Living with diabetes can be hard enough, but traveling can really complicate things. Don't stay home for fear of being without your medicine or not finding the right food when you need it. People with diabetes can travel for fun or commute to a job — as long as they plan ahead and follow these simple steps.

5 easy ways to combat diabetes

The American Diabetes Association offers new eating advice for people with diabetes. Follow these rules to maintain a healthy weight, control your blood sugar, and avoid dangerous complications.

▸ Eat more healthy carbohydrates, like fruits, vegetables, legumes, low-fat milk, and whole grains.

▸ Limit saturated fats to less than 7 percent of your total calories. You'll find them in meat, egg yolks, whole milk, butter, cream, and cheese.

▸ Avoid trans fats. Check package labels to find where trans fats lurk.

▸ Cut cholesterol to less than 200 milligrams a day.

▸ Eat fish at least twice a week. Make it baked, broiled, or blackened, but not fried.

Carry plenty of supplies. Some people carry at least five days' worth of extra supplies for blood sugar testing or insulin injections — no matter where they go. You can usually purchase supplies for the lowest price when you use your insurance benefits at certain drugstores. If you don't plan ahead and have to buy emergency supplies, you could pay a lot more.

Don't skip exercise. If you drive a long way to work or spend lots of time in airports or on trains, you may have trouble fitting exercise into your schedule. Make time on your lunch hour for walking, or take some laps around the airport terminal while you wait for your flight.

Seek out the best food options. Eating in a restaurant can be tricky, but many offer low-fat or other healthy meal options. Some chain restaurants carry nutritional information on their Web sites, so you can see your options before you arrive. Carry extra rations, like Glucerna Meal Bars or DiabetX Snack Bars, in case there's nothing on the menu that will work. In a pinch, stop by a grocery store for whole-grain bread and peanut butter or cheese.

Keep snacks in your car. Dangers of hypoglycemia, or low blood sugar, increase if you have to drive. Low blood sugar can make you feel weak and fatigued, and it also impairs your thinking and eyesight. Know your own warning signs, and carry plenty of glucose tablets or snacks with you. Don't assume you'll be able to find a snack when you travel.

Pack supplies in your carry-on bag. Although airport security has become more strict, you can take your insulin, syringes, glucose-testing supplies — even lancets and needles — on an airplane. Prescription medication must have a professionally printed label identifying the medication and manufacturer's name or a pharmaceutical label. The prescription medicine must match the name on the passenger's ticket. The Transportation Security Administration (TSA) also allows people with diabetes and similar medical conditions to carry glucose gel packets, tablets, or other sugar sources to use in case of low blood sugar.

Protect your drugs. Don't leave insulin, other drugs, and testing strips in a hot car, and don't pack them in a suitcase to be checked on an airplane. Too much heat or cold can damage drugs, especially liquids. It can also harm testing strips. Carry your fragile supplies in an insulated bag, and never leave it in a hot car.

9 ways to keep your feet healthy

Each year almost 73,000 people have lower limb amputations because of problems related to diabetes. In fact, aside from accidents, diabetes is the main cause of foot amputations.

About a third of all people with diabetes suffer from neuropathy, or nerve damage. Neuropathy can make your feet unable to feel heat, cold, or pain. You could step on a tack and not even feel it. High blood sugar can damage your blood vessels, causing circulation problems. If this happens, cuts, scrapes, or blisters can take a long time to heal and become infected. Eventually, the infection can spread to your bones.

Treating the bone infection, called osteomyelitis, requires a trip to the hospital and costs about $35,000. About 8 percent of people with osteomyelitis have a foot or leg amputated, 23 percent a toe.

The best way to avoid problems is to pay attention to your feet. Follow these suggestions from the American Diabetes Association to keep your feet healthy.

▶ Inspect your feet daily for cuts, blisters, sores, or swelling. Get someone to help you or use a mirror if you can't see the bottoms of your feet.

▶ Have your feet checked by your doctor at least once a year — more often if you have had foot problems.

▶ Get in the habit of wiggling your toes and flexing your ankles while you sit to improve circulation. Don't cross your legs when you sit. This keeps blood from flowing freely to your legs and feet.

Where to find free eye care

Poor control of your blood sugar can damage the small blood vessels in your retina and lead to blurred vision and blindness. This complication of diabetes, called diabetic retinopathy, is the most common cause of blindness in adults, making people with diabetes 25 times more likely to become blind than other people. An eye doctor can see the problem by dilating your eye and looking at your retina.

EyeCare America offers free exams and one year of care for people with diabetes. You must be at least 65 years old and a U.S. citizen or legal resident. Also, you can't be receiving health care through an HMO or the Veterans Administration. For more information, go online to *aao.org/eyecare-america*.

▶ Call your doctor if you have an ingrown toenail, numbness, or pain, or if you see a change in skin color.

▶ Wash and dry your feet carefully every day. To prevent dry skin, use a lotion on the tops and bottoms of your feet.

▶ Cut your toenails straight across, but file down sharp corners that might cut the next toe.

▶ Never go barefoot, even in your house. Keep slippers by your bed to avoid bumping into things at night.

▶ Wear shoes that fit well and don't rub. Check the insides of your shoes for bumps, tears, or other places that could cause trouble.

▶ Wear socks that are soft and thick enough for extra protection. Choose material that will draw moisture away from your skin, like acrylic.

If you have diabetes and a history of foot ulcers or amputation, you may be eligible for help. Medicare will pay 80 percent of the cost of specially prescribed shoes and inserts under its Part B coverage.

Flu

Low-cost prevention is your best option

If you think the flu is just an overblown cold, think again. More than 200,000 people are hospitalized and about 36,000 die every year from influenza and related complications. Although it begins like a cold, the flu quickly knocks you off your feet. Suddenly your head hurts, your body aches, you have a fever, and you're so tired you can barely move. The virus can spread quickly, too, especially when people are in close contact.

Your annual flu shot goes a long way toward keeping you well, but it's not a guarantee. People over the age of 65 have the highest risk and are more likely to fall victim to pneumonia and other bacterial infections. Complications like these may develop when you're weak from the flu, and chronic illnesses like heart disease, asthma, and diabetes can get worse.

It doesn't cost much to keep yourself safe. As the old adage says, "an ounce of prevention is worth a pound of cure."

Beat the flu with smart protection

An annual flu vaccine is the best thing you can do to prevent the flu. You build up immunity to the virus when your body reacts to killed viruses in the vaccine. It's important to get one every year because flu viruses constantly change, and fresh vaccines meet the challenge of new and different bugs.

But flu protection does not have to cost you a fortune. For starters, your employer or local health department may offer free flu vaccinations. Medicare Part B and some other insurance plans also will pay for it. You can get a flu shot from your doctor, the health department, or other health care provider. Private health-care companies also set up clinics in grocery stores, drugstores, and other locations. Look on the Web site *vaccinefinder.org/find-vaccine* for a list of places that offer flu shots.

Flu shots are safe for anyone older than six months unless they have a severe allergy to chicken eggs, are running a fever, or experienced a previous reaction to the vaccine. Groups especially encouraged to get a flu shot every year include:

▶ people over 50 years old and those with certain chronic medical conditions.

▶ people living in nursing homes or similar facilities.

Second shot knocks out pneumonia

While you're getting your flu shot, roll up the sleeve on your other arm and get a pneumonia shot, too. The pneumococcal polysaccharide vaccine (PPV) protects you against 23 kinds of pneumococcal bacteria, including some that lead to pneumonia, a serious complication of the flu.

Pneumococcal diseases are now more resistant to penicillin and other drugs that used to control them, so it's important to prevent them through vaccination. Everyone over age 65, as well as younger people with health problems, should have a PPV shot.

- children under 5 years old.

- caregivers for people with high influenza risk, including those listed above and children less than six months old.

The Centers for Disease Control and Prevention (CDC) recommends people get a flu shot by the end of October, but you can still get vaccinated later since the flu season sometimes lasts until May. It takes about two weeks for the protective antibodies to kick in, and protection peaks in four to six weeks. The vaccine will work faster if you've previously had a flu shot or the flu itself.

Flu vaccine also comes in a nasal spray instead of a shot, but it is only approved for healthy people between 2 and 49 years old who are not pregnant.

You can't get influenza from a flu shot, but it may cause aches, a low-grade fever, or a sore arm. These side effects go away in a day or two.

Recent research has shown the flu vaccine may not be as effective for older people as once thought. But it still offers significant protection, so don't be tempted to skip it. If you get the flu in spite of the shot, it won't be as bad and you'll likely avoid serious complications like pneumonia, hospitalization, and death.

6 secrets to staying healthy

A healthy lifestyle is important if you want to avoid the flu. By keeping your body in top shape, you have a better chance of fighting off illness. The same formula you follow to head off a cold works wonders for the flu, too.

- Wash your hands often. You can pick up viruses from any contaminated object, including doorknobs and telephones.

- Stay away from crowds and people who appear sick. The flu virus spreads in tiny droplets tossed into the air from coughing and sneezing.

- Eat a healthy diet. Include yogurt with immune-boosting live cultures and whole-grain cereals full of selenium.

- Drink lots of fluids. They keep your throat lining moist and supple so it won't crack and let viruses in.

- Get plenty of rest. It builds up your resistance to illness and helps your whole system stay in balance.

- Quit smoking, if you need to. It raises your risk for respiratory infections. Avoid air pollution and second-hand smoke, too.

A little stress may boost your flu shot. Women in a British study who exercised physically or mentally just before getting the shot produced more flu antibodies.

Missed your flu shot? Vitamin D to the rescue

Most flu outbreaks happen in the winter when people aren't getting much vitamin D from the sun. Researchers don't think that's a coincidence. Vitamin D actually boosts your immune system and helps you fight off infections like the flu. One way it does this is by amping up natural antibiotics in your body that wipe out invading germs.

To make up for those short winter days, eat more vitamin D foods like salmon, sardines, mushrooms, and fortified cereals and milk. Or take a supplement of at least 600 international units (IU) a day.

Easy clues to the flu

Symptom	Flu	Cold
extreme exhaustion	usual, early, often severe	never
fever	usual, high (102-104 degrees F), lasts 3-4 days	rare
general aches, pains	usual, often severe	slight, maybe not at all
fatigue, weakness	usual, can last 2-3 weeks	possible, but mild
headache	almost always	rare
chest discomfort, cough	common, can be severe	mild to moderate, hacking cough
sneezing	sometimes	usual
stuffy nose	sometimes	common
sore throat	sometimes	common

Source: National Institute of Allergy and Infectious Diseases

Mission critical — stop flu virus with secret weapon

Your body is primed and ready to fight off all kinds of attacks. But the flu virus is like a ninja — cloaked in a special protein that lets it slip into your cells before your immune system knows it's there.

Fortunately, you can call on a secret agent to break up mucus, open sinuses, and fight germs — tea. The best part? It's made from three pantry staples.

▸ Green tea. It's loaded with catechins, phytochemicals that barricade influenza's entry into cells. In one study, children who drank 1 to 5 cups of green tea daily cut their risk of getting the flu. In another study, researchers gave adults green tea capsules equaling 10 cups of tea daily for three months. Fewer got sick compared to the placebo group, and those who did weren't sick as long.

▸ Honey. Nerve fibers that trigger cough are near the nerve fibers that help you taste sweetness. Researchers think these may interact when you eat honey and give you an advantage in subduing a rogue cough. And honey's got the World Health Organization's approval for this mission. To get more antioxidants, go with the darker varieties.

▸ Turmeric. Call in this powerful condiment to elude the flu. Turmeric's curcumin — an antioxidant-of-all-trades — fights several viral, bacterial, and fungal foes, including influenza in one test tube study.

Here are two ways to secure the benefits of honey turmeric green tea.

Prepare it hot to soothe sinuses. Brew your tea for four minutes on low heat, around 167 degrees. The low temp will help preserve the catechins and flavor. For each cup, stir in up to 1/4 teaspoon of ground, grated, or powdered turmeric, and add honey to taste. Then breathe in the steam and drink it warm to let the water vapor tickle your irritated sinuses and stimulate mucus flow.

Mucus cleans and protects your sinuses. It thickens when you're sick, which can make you more miserable. Because bacteria cling to mucus, encouraging your nose to run means you get rid of both faster.

Cool it to take out more germs. To get even more flu-fighting compounds, steep 4 teaspoons of loose tea leaves or three tea bags in a quart of water in the refrigerator for 12 hours.

A study of brewing methods revealed a higher level of antioxidants from this cold-brew technique for two reasons. First, the tea leaves are in the water longer, allowing more of the good compounds to infuse the drink. Second, the low temperature protects the beneficial compounds that can break down in higher temps.

Don't want to wait? Brewing tea over low heat for five minutes then quickly icing it is nearly as effective as the cold-brew method. The rapid cooling protects compounds from long exposure to harsh, high temperatures. Plus you can stir in the honey when it's still warm to help it dissolve easier.

Feel better with 3 natural flu fighters

Many people prefer natural remedies to fight the flu. If you would rather rely on non-drug solutions, here are three you should consider. They're not guaranteed to work, but they won't hurt you and there is strong support for each of them.

Elderberry. The flowers and berries of this ancient bush have been used for centuries as folk cures. Scientific research suggests the extract may be an effective remedy for the flu. In a study of 60 Norwegians, flu symptoms went away an average of four days quicker for those who took Sambucol, an elderberry syrup product. The leaves and stems of the elder tree are toxic, so look for commercially prepared elderberry extracts in liquid, capsule, or tablet form.

> What many people call the "stomach flu" is not influenza but gastroenteritis, caused by other viruses, bacteria, or toxins.

Astragalus. This Chinese medicine staple strengthens your immune system, say its supporters. It particularly increases resistance to viruses and is a great source of the powerful antioxidant selenium. It comes in many forms, but herbalists prefer to use it as a tincture. Take astragalus long-term for prevention of colds and flu rather than waiting until you are sick.

Sauerkraut. Korean scientists say *lactobacilli* bacteria, which give fermented cabbage its tangy sourness, have antiviral powers. In a recent study, they cured chickens infected with bird flu by feeding them kimchi, Korea's national cabbage dish. And no reports of bird flu in humans have surfaced in Korea or Japan, where kimchi is also popular. Sauerkraut, another fermented cabbage product, has the same protective power, say the scientists.

> Don't be too quick to bring fever down. It's your body's natural defense against flu viruses, which die off when body temperatures rise above normal.

Flu fighters from the sea

Next winter, give yourself a better shot at avoiding the flu. Eat some seaweed. *Undaria pinnatifida*, which wakame and mekabu come from, is rich in fucoidan, a compound that fights inflammation and possibly viruses.

Seniors who ate fucoidan sprinkled on their lunches every day had more virus-fighting immune cells than seniors who didn't eat seaweed sprinkles. They also had a stronger immune reaction to the flu shot. That's a good thing. It means the vaccine worked better and made them less likely to catch the flu.

Flu vaccines don't protect you as well when you're older because your immune system weakens with age. Goose yours into higher gear by eating a quarter cup of seaweed salad made from wakame, or a small side of mekabu. You can also buy granules made from brown seaweeds and use them in place of table salt.

Dollars&Sense
Get free drugs the easy way

You could save hundreds of dollars with free prescription drugs including virtually every brand name available. You might even nab extra savings from free over-the-counter drugs. You just need to know where to look.

Claim your prescription freebies. Drug companies constantly shower doctors with free samples of prescription drugs to hand out to patients like you. So don't hesitate to ask your doctor for free drug samples anytime she writes a prescription. Samples can save you money in ways you might not expect.

For example, you'll have time to comparison shop for the best prices until your samples run out. Finding the cheapest source for your medicine could lead to years of savings. Moreover, prescription drug samples are a golden opportunity to road test a drug that is new to you. You won't lose a dime if the drug causes unbearable side effects or turns out to be ineffective.

Try over-the-counter drugs for free. You could also nab free samples of over-the-counter medications, like Metamucil, Motrin IB, Tylenol P.M., Alka-Seltzer, and more. Check with your doctor first, especially if she recommends the medicine. Drug companies are not limited to giving out prescription samples, so your doctor may have nonprescription freebies, too.

If your doctor does not have free samples, consider these options.

▸ Visit the product's Web site. Although some sites may not currently offer free giveaways, you could still find money-saving coupons.

▸ Visit *www.all-free-samples.com*. Click the "Health" link to see current offerings of free drug samples.

Gallstones

Sound strategies for a healthy gallbladder

About 700,000 people have their gallbladders removed every year, but you don't have to be one of them. Here's how you can keep your gallbladder healthy and prevent troublesome gallstones.

Gallstones start with bile, a fluid made in your liver that helps digest fat. Bile is a valuable mix of water, cholesterol, fat, salt, bilirubin, and protein, and it's stored in your gallbladder. Stones can form if too much cholesterol, bile salts, or bilirubin builds up in your bile and stagnates in your gallbladder. Many stones can develop, or just one. They can be as small as a grain of sand or as large as an egg. But even a small stone can cause trouble.

When bile is needed to help digest a meal, your gallbladder squeezes it into your intestines through tiny tubes called ducts. If a stone creates a blockage in a duct, it can cause inflammation, infection, and pain. People who have frequent problems may decide to have surgery to remove the gallbladder.

Slash risk with one easy trick

Here's a cheap and easy way to reduce your risk of gallstones — take a walk. Women who did the least walking had a 59-percent greater risk of gallstone disease than women who walked the most, a recent

University of Pittsburgh study reports. Not surprisingly, exercise doesn't just work for women. Men can gain protection, too.

But walking isn't your only option. You can choose a different activity, like swimming, biking, or dancing. As long as you get moving, you're on the right track. And if you burn up some calories and fat, you might lower your gallstone risk even more.

Aim for two to three hours of exercise every week. Some chores count as exercise, too. According to the Calorie Control Council, the following chart shows how many calories a 150-pound person would burn by doing a particular activity for just 30 minutes.

Slash gallstone risk with household chores

Activities	Calories burned
Scrubbing floors	189
Raking	171
Gardening	162
Mowing the lawn	162
Washing a car	153
Walking a dog	149
Grocery shopping	122
Vacuuming	85

The danger of crash diets

Being overweight significantly raises your gallstone risk, especially if you carry extra weight around your middle. In fact, research shows that women with bigger waists are more likely to have gall-bladder removal surgery.

Fortunately, weight around your middle is the easiest kind to lose. Getting rid of it may lower your risk for heart disease and diabetes, as well as gallstones. Here's how it works.

Scientists have discovered that deep abdominal fat, the kind that wraps around your liver and other organs, can trigger gallstones and other health problems. Moreover, extra pounds make your liver churn out extra cholesterol, raising your odds of developing gall-stones even more.

You'll lower your risk by losing inches around your waist, often before you lose pounds. If you don't have much fat around your waist, you can still cut your chances of developing gallstones by reaching and maintaining a healthy weight.

Here's something else to remember — forget starvation diets when you are trying to lose weight. Scientists say rapid weight loss, crash diets, or repeatedly losing and regaining weight will make your liver produce extra cholesterol. Gallstones develop in a sur-prising number of people who lose weight quickly. Instead, talk with your doctor about a sensible weight loss plan. If she recommends rapid weight loss for health reasons, she can prescribe medication to help dissolve any small gallstones that form.

Otherwise, stick to a healthy diet and exercise regularly to lose one or two pounds

Some herbs can be dangerous to use if you have gallstones. Talk to your doctor before using artichoke leaf, turmeric, dandelion, and ginger.

a week. It's far cheaper than stone-dissolving treatments, and you may discover new dishes and activities you'll wish you'd uncovered years ago.

Simple ways to stop stones cold

The next time you're at the grocery store, spend more time in the produce aisle. Foods that grew up in a sunny field or orchard can help you fight gallstones. Try these super suggestions, too.

Eat more fiber. Fruits and vegetables, hearty whole-grain breads and cereals, and delicious seeds and nuts are all fierce gallstone fighters thanks to their fiber. When you don't get enough fiber, your body reabsorbs too much cholesterol. That excess cholesterol can form gallstones if it gets into bile.

However, soluble fiber absorbs cholesterol-loaded bile in your intestines and sweeps it out of your body. Enjoy oranges, oats, barley, beans, and asparagus to get more soluble fiber.

After gallbladder surgery, keeping tabs on your cholesterol may be more important than it was before. Get your cholesterol checked regularly.

Insoluble fiber helps cut bile production and keep digestive products moving. It also reduces other risk factors for gallstones. Rich sources of insoluble fiber include brown rice, whole grains, wheat bran, seeds, beans, and popcorn. Most fruits and veggies contain both kinds of fiber.

Boost vitamin C intake. Researchers found less gallbladder disease in women who had high blood levels of vitamin C. They've also linked deficiency in this vitamin to a higher risk of gallstones. Scientists think vitamin C may help break down the cholesterol in bile. So add more pineapple, papaya, and oranges and other citrus fruits and juices to your diet. Or try tasty foods like sweet peppers, strawberries, kiwi, frozen peaches, and broccoli.

Watch the carbs. A recent study shows that people who eat lots of carbohydrates, including bread, cereal, sugar, and starchy vegetables like potatoes, have a higher risk for gallstones. A high-carbohydrate diet increases insulin production, which can boost your cholesterol. The researchers recommend avoiding high-carbohydrate, low-fat diets. If you eat too little fat, the gallbladder won't contract and empty its bile. You need a meal with about 10 grams of fat for the gallbladder to contract normally.

> In a study of 800 women, those who ate meat were twice as likely to develop gallstones as the vegetarians.

Choose fantastic fats. Eat the same healthy fats as the Greeks, and you might avoid your own personal Stone Age. Research suggests that the unsaturated fats found in the Mediterranean diet may fight gallstones.

▸ Enjoy peanuts, walnuts, almonds, and even peanut butter. Harvard researchers discovered that women who ate the most nuts had 25-percent less risk of gallbladder removal surgery than women who avoided nuts or rarely ate them.

▸ Choose olive oil, canola oil, flaxseed, and the omega-3 fatty acids in fish to lower your gallstone risk. If you are worried about mercury and other toxins in fish, choose these varieties — salmon, herring, sardines, mackerel, and flounder. And only eat fish twice a week.

▸ Limit or avoid meats, butter, whole milk, cheese, fried foods, stick margarine, and packaged foods that contain trans fatty acids or saturated fat. New research shows trans fatty acids can raise gallstone risk in men. What's more, too much saturated fat slows digestion and raises cholesterol, the main ingredient in most gallstones.

Brew news: Coffee stalls gallstone buildup

"What goes best with a cup of coffee? Another cup," joked Henry Rollins, an American comedian. And when it comes to preventing gallstones, he's right on the money.

Coffee's perks are well-grounded. Drinking just 1 cup of coffee each day decreases your risk of developing gallstones by 5 percent. Up your intake by 1 more cup, and you'll see even better results.

Researchers discovered that folks who drink 2 cups of caffeinated coffee every day reduce their risk of gallbladder disease by 11 percent. Have 3 cups, and your risk drops by 15 percent. If you're a real coffee buff, you might even indulge in as many as 4 cups a day. If so, your caffeine habit could be the ticket to lower your risk of developing gallstones by nearly 20 percent. Great news for coffee lovers, but how's it work?

Stonewall gallstones with a gut reaction. Scientists think it may be the caffeine in coffee that stimulates the contraction of the gallbladder. This helps get rid of the cholesterol-filled bile that can harden into stones. So coffee is good news for preventing gallstones — and for keeping small crystals from turning into bigger ones.

But researchers are stumped. If it were just the caffeine at work, caffeinated sodas or teas would have the same effect. Oops. They don't. So, although caffeine helps, there's a mystery ingredient in coffee that's warding off those stones.

If coffee's not your cup of tea, wet your whistle with water instead. H2O helps your gallbladder empty so bile can't build up. And that prevents gallstones from forming. Researchers think 2 cups of water, four times a day should keep your gallbladder humming along right as rain.

Experts think it may be coffee's magnesium. One study showed that men who got adequate amounts of magnesium in their diets — that's 420 milligrams (mg) per day for men and 320 mg for women — had a 32 percent lower risk of developing gallstones than their magnesium-deficient peers. More magnesium research is needed, but for now, relax and enjoy a healthy cuppa joe — it's good to the last drop.

Don't ignore gallstones

Don't be tempted to ignore gallbladder problems. Stones can block bile flow if they lodge in the ducts that carry it from the liver to the small intestine. If ducts remain blocked for long, you can suffer severe damage or infection to your gallbladder, liver, or pancreas. Warning signs include fever, jaundice, and persistent pain.

Strike back at gallstone attack

Take these steps to cut your risk of painful gallstones.

Avoid HRT pills. If you're a woman thinking about hormone-replacement therapy (HRT), consider using a patch or cream form rather than a pill. One study found a lower risk of gallstones among women taking HRT through the skin rather than oral therapy.

Oral HRT may raise your risk of gallstones because the hormones are broken down in your liver before they enter your bloodstream. In contrast, hormones you absorb through your skin move directly into your blood, avoiding this "first-pass metabolism" in the liver.

Experts say for every 140 women who choose patch or cream HRT over pills for five years, one gallbladder removal is avoided.

See about statins. To reduce the risk of gallstones that need surgery, ask your doctor about taking a statin — especially if you have high cholesterol or other risk factors for heart disease.

Researchers in England found that middle-age people who took a statin for at least a year had a lower risk of gallstones needing surgery. Similarly, women in the Nurses' Health Study who took cholesterol-lowering drugs — mostly statins — had less risk of gallbladder removal.

What's the connection? Statins keep your liver from making too much cholesterol, and gallstones are made of either bilirubin or cholesterol. Less cholesterol in your system means less cholesterol that can be made into gallstones.

GERD

Low-cost and no-cost solutions for heartburn

Americans spend around $10 billion a year on prescription drugs to fight gastroesophageal reflux disease (GERD). If you're one of the 60 million people who get heartburn, you might have GERD, too.

When you eat, food passes through your esophagus to your stomach, where hydrochloric acid and other juices break down the food. To keep this powerful acid out of your esophagus, a valve at the top of your stomach closes. This valve is called the lower esophageal sphincter (LES), and it only relaxes to let food into your stomach. But if the LES relaxes when it shouldn't, stomach acid splashes up into your esophagus. This is called reflux.

Frequent reflux can irritate the lining of your esophagus leading to serious damage. About 10 to 15 percent of GERD cases turn into Barrett's esophagus, a condition linked to esophageal cancer. Only about one in five people with this cancer live five years or longer after diagnosis.

10 tricks to tame heartburn

Even if you've never been overweight, moderate weight gain could make your GERD symptoms worse, a recent study suggests. Researchers found that women at a healthy weight who gained a modest amount of weight also gained an extra risk of nagging symptoms.

On top of that, your odds for GERD and esophageal cancer can double when you're overweight. Extra pounds put pressure on your stomach area, which can loosen the LES and send digestive juices into your esophagus. Lose weight and you might lose your GERD symptoms, too.

In fact, why take Nexium when there are easy, no-cost solutions for acid reflux. Try these inexpensive tips and tricks before you take your chances with dangerous medicine.

End nightly heartburn. Sleep on your left side for relief that really works. Your esophagus angles slightly to the left where it connects to your stomach. So when you rest on your left side, acid faces a tough uphill climb to reach your esophagus. A sleeping wedge behind your back may keep you facing left.

Take advantage of acid's "low tide." Give stomach acid time to dwindle. Don't eat for at least two hours before bedtime and don't lie down for at least two hours after eating.

Delay after-dinner activity. Wait 90 minutes after eating before starting any strenuous exercise.

Avoid straining. Heavy lifting and straining makes your abdominal muscles contract and squeeze stomach acid into your esophagus.

Ease the pressure. Wear clothes and belts that fit comfortably around your stomach. Give away anything that's too tight.

Sit up straight when you eat. Never stand, lie down, or bend over after eating. This drives food and stomach acid back up into your esophagus.

Get help from gravity. Let gravity pull the contents of your stomach away from your esophagus so you can sleep. Place blocks under your bedposts to raise the head of your bed about 6 inches, or tuck a sleeping wedge under your mattress.

When to call for help

Signs that your chest pain is something more serious than heart-burn include nausea, sweating, weakness, breathlessness, fainting, or shooting pain from your jaw to your arm. If you experience one or more of these symptoms, you might be having a heart attack. Call 911 or ask someone to drive you to the hospital.

Tame tablet trouble. Make pills go down and stay down. Take medications with plenty of water, and don't lie down after swallowing a pill.

Stop carrying a torch. Nicotine boosts acid production and relaxes the LES, allowing stomach acid to creep into your esophagus. Although saliva washes the acid back out of your esophagus, smoking decreases saliva, too. Find a way to quit to ease your symptoms.

Get both sides of the alcohol story. Large amounts of alcohol can irritate the lining of your esophagus. Combine that with smoking and you may raise your risk of deadly esophageal cancer. However, a recent study suggests that a small amount of alcohol may protect the esophageal lining. Just don't forget that drinking alcoholic beverages still increases stomach acid and relaxes the LES.

Fight fire with food

Guess what may be back on the menu if you have GERD — chocolate, spicy foods, orange juice, and coffee. Eliminating these foods may not help heartburn or other GERD symptoms, according to a new study.

But the study's researchers say this might not apply to everyone. In fact, another study showed that 44 percent of people with GERD symptoms saw improvement after changing their diets. So here's your best bet. Keep a detailed diary of the foods you eat, when you eat them, when your heartburn occurs and when it doesn't. Pay special attention to these heartburn triggers.

- citrus fruits and juices — orange, lemon, lime, and grapefruit
- foods and drinks containing peppermint or spearmint
- chocolate
- tomato products, including ketchup
- mustard, pepper, onions, garlic, and vinegar
- high-fat foods, especially foods high in saturated fat
- greasy or spicy foods
- beverages that contain caffeine
- carbonated beverages

Hypochlorhydria — a condition in which your stomach doesn't produce enough acid — can actually cause a number of GERD symptoms. Your doctor can run tests to determine if this is the cause of your reflux symptoms.

Soon you'll know which foods trigger trouble and which ones don't. You can also unleash more weapons against GERD and cancer with these dietary secrets.

Strike back with fiber. The more fiber you get, the lower your risk of GERD symptoms. So enjoy more whole grains and low-acid fruits and vegetables. Not only can whole grains help soak up extra stomach acid, but selenium-rich whole grain products may help defend against dangerous cell changes in Barrett's esophagus.

Treat yourself to green tea. You may have less chance of getting esophageal cancer if you drink green tea often, studies suggest. Polyphenols, antioxidants found in tea, may be the reason why.

Green tea has the most polyphenols, followed closely by black and oolong teas.

Make water your ally. Water rinses acid out of your esophagus and dilutes the acid in your stomach. Aim for six to eight 8-ounce glasses daily. In fact, try drinking small amounts of water throughout the day. Drinking too much at once could distend your stomach and rev up your heartburn. And don't drink liquids with meals or you might not get enough stomach acid to digest your food. Stop drinking an hour before and resume an hour after eating.

Pass on processed meats. The nitrates and chemicals in these meats may raise the risk of esophageal cancer in people with GERD.

Encourage easier swallowing. If you have trouble swallowing, avoid tough meats, vegetables with skins, and pasta.

Stop overeating. Large meals raise acid production, and a full stomach is more likely to spill over into your esophagus.

Uncover the cause of your heartburn

Antacids and over-the-counter versions of prescription drugs may suppress symptoms while GERD stealthily wreaks more damage. If heartburn bothers you twice a week or more, see your doctor. He can check your esophagus for damage and uncover what's causing your symptoms.

Beware of heartburn-free GERD

Even if you don't have heartburn, you might still have GERD. Constantly clearing your throat is a symptom of GERD. So are these.

▶ trouble swallowing   ▶ sore throat

- chest pain ▸ abdominal pain
- the feeling that something is stuck in your throat

Other surprising signs that you may have GERD — with or without heartburn — include a hoarse voice, chronic cough, erosion of your tooth enamel, breathing difficulty in people who have asthma, and lung disease. If you have these symptoms, see your doctor.

Good news for coffee lovers

You enjoy drinking coffee, but not the heartburn that follows. Switching to a dark-roasted coffee could help. Researchers discovered that dark-roasted coffee contains a compound that helps reduce stomach acid.

Called N-methylpyridinium (NMP), this compound is generated only with roasting. So dark-roasted coffee contains more of it — up to twice as much as light-roasted varieties. Unlike NMP, caffeine helps stimulate the secretion of stomach acid. So a decaffeinated, dark-roasted coffee might be your best bet.

Got GERD? Tap into turmeric's healing powers

No doubt about it. Turmeric will add a glorious shade of gold to your tasty curries and stews. But this aromatic spice's powers don't stop there. Long valued as a traditional medicine, natural compounds in turmeric have been found to slow unwanted hair growth, cleanse wounds, and help neutralize deadly cobra venom.

One of those compounds — a polyphenol called curcumin — acts as a strong antioxidant and anti-inflammatory. Those powers may prove essential in the treatment of gastroesophageal reflux disease (GERD).

One study designed to mimic the effects of stomach acid backwash on people with GERD found that curcumin blocked cytokine activity in esophageal cells. How does that help? Cytokines are powerful proteins known to cause inflammation.

Scientists also looked at how curcumin might help people with Barrett's esophagus — a condition in which GERD causes abnormal cellular changes to the lining of the lower esophagus. Those changes are thought to increase the risk of developing cancer.

The researchers found that a daily dose of 500 milligrams of curcumin over seven days doubled the frequency of apoptosis — that is, the rate at which dysfunctional cells die on schedule — in people with Barrett's esophagus.

Why is that good? One of the hallmarks of cancer is the ability of abnormal cells to evade apoptosis, divide without control, and invade surrounding tissue or spread to other parts of the body.

A low-carb diet relieves GERD symptoms

Some experts think a low-carb diet can help GERD symptoms and reduce acids. This may be because protein and fat take longer to digest, which gives stomach acid something else to do besides sneak back into your esophagus.

Generally, a low-carb diet includes meat, poultry, fish, eggs, and vegetables like asparagus, broccoli, carrots, squash, and cucumbers. Avoid eating a lot of legumes, fruits, breads, sweets, pastas, and starchy vegetables, like corn, peas, and potatoes.

A study published in *Digestive Diseases and Sciences* supports the low-carb diet. The meal plan included less than 20 grams of carbohydrates a day, but you should talk to your doctor first to discuss the best eating plan for you.

Put heartburn to rest with melatonin

Suffering from heartburn? Melatonin may provide relief. You probably think of melatonin as the sleep hormone, but it also plays an important role in digestive health. In fact, evidence suggests that melatonin may be an effective treatment for gastroesophageal reflux disease (GERD) — with fewer side effects than commonly prescribed drugs.

In one study, a Brazilian researcher compared a combination of melatonin and other nutrients to omeprazole, a proton pump inhibitor often used to treat GERD symptoms. The supplement included 6 milligrams (mg) of melatonin, plus tryptophan, vitamin B6, vitamin B12, methionine, folic acid, and betaine.

Some say it's bad luck to spill salt. But shaking it on your food? A study of 25,562 adults in a Norwegian public health survey found that those who added table salt to their meals ran a 70 percent higher risk of acid reflux than those who never did so.

After 40 days, all 176 people in the melatonin group reported relief of symptoms, compared to just two-thirds of those in the omeprazole group. After the study, the 60 people in the omeprazole group who did not respond to the drug switched to the melatonin blend for 40 days — and all of them found relief.

Melatonin may work by preventing the secretion of stomach acid and by stopping the lower esophageal sphincter, the valve between the stomach and esophagus, from relaxing at the wrong time.

The recommended amount to soothe heartburn is 6 mg of melatonin taken around bedtime. Experts suggest sticking with your normal GERD medications for the first 40 days of melatonin treatment. After that, keep a dose of your regular medication on hand, and take it whenever symptoms reappear. If you are taking a prescription drug to relieve your symptoms, check with your doctor before trying melatonin.

2 ways to fight a deadly complication of GERD

GERD, Barrett's esophagus, and esophageal cancer have a lot in common. If you leave gastroesophageal reflux disease (GERD) untreated, you could be faced with serious complications such as Barrett's esophagus or esophageal cancer.

Here are some foods that help keep your esophagus healthy.

Vanquish Barrett's with antioxidant-packed veggies. Good news for veggie lovers — dark green, leafy green, raw, and cruciferous vegetables are full of nutrients that may protect against cancer. Eat more foods like broccoli, cabbage, collard greens, kale, spinach, and mustard greens. They're packed with vitamin C and beta carotene — antioxidants that may help combat the damaging effects of GERD and reduce your risk of developing Barrett's esophagus and esophageal cancer.

Give yourself a boost with cancer-fighting berries. Berries are superstar fruits you can use to perk up a salad, jazz up a dessert, or revive a frozen treat. Nutritionists call them superfruits because they are loaded with cancer-fighting antioxidants and nutrients, including vitamins A, C, and E, folic acid, selenium, calcium, beta carotene, lutein, and several anthocyanins.

In one animal study published in *Nutrition and Cancer*, black raspberries, strawberries, and blackberries blocked the growth of tumors by 24 to 56 percent within 25 weeks compared to the animals that didn't eat berries.

Anxiety and stress can bring on heartburn, but regular exercise is a champion stress fighter. Battle stress and heartburn at the same time by being more active.

Chewing gum — simple way to stick it to heartburn

Scientific studies show smacking on a stick of gum could relieve heartburn as well as, or better than, antacids. Chewing regular or sugar-free gum stimulates the flow of saliva, which contains natural antacids. This extra spit neutralizes the acid that has leaked into your esophagus, the cause of that uncomfortable, burning feeling, and washes it back down to your stomach.

A small but significant clinical trial shows chewing a stick of gum after meals may counteract acid reflux. Researchers studied 12 people with gastroesophageal reflux disease (GERD) and 24 people without GERD. Chewing gum for an hour after eating lowered the amount of acid in the esophagus of GERD sufferers for three hours. Since acid reflux usually occurs within three hours of eating, these experts say gum lasts long enough to manage after-meal reflux.

If that sounds good, get ready for even more relief. A few manufacturers now make gum containing an antacid such as calcium carbonate, the active ingredient in Tums. This combines the power of an antacid tablet with your body's own saliva, boosting gum's power to put out the flames.

In fact, antacid gum may relieve heartburn faster and for a longer time than regular gum or antacid alone. Experts at the Oklahoma Foundation for Digestive Research gave volunteers a high-dose antacid gum, low-dose antacid gum, chewable antacid tablet, or placebo.

Both the high- and low-dose gums soothed heartburn and neutralized acid in the esophagus better than placebo. They eased discomfort for at least two hours after meals, and both worked faster and provided longer-lasting relief than the antacid tablet alone.

Dollars&Sense
Order up amazing drug bargains

Slash the high cost of prescriptions, and discover where to get the best deals, legally, safely, and best of all, cheaply.

Order meds by mail. Now everyone can save with AARP Prescription Discounts. This discount program is available to everyone, whether you are an AARP member or not. Visit *aarp-pharmacy.com* or call 877-422-7718 for information to get started.

Cut drug prices by heading online. You can save money and get your prescriptions delivered right to your door by shopping online. Internet pharmacies have fewer costs than drugstores, so they often offer better prescription discounts.

Keep in mind, drug prices can vary dramatically, even online. Fortunately, there's a reputable Web site to help take the guesswork out of comparison shopping.

You can check out prescription drug prices at a variety of internet pharmacies with a single click of your mouse at *pharmacy checker.com*. The little-known site also researches mail order and internet pharmacies, then ranks them by safety and online security, among other criteria.

Wherever you shop, watch out for expensive shipping and handling charges. These quickly add up, turning a fantastic bargain into an expensive nightmare.

Avoid online dangers. You can use your computer to get the very best price on your prescriptions, but you must also know which pharmacies you should never get a prescription from. After all, some sites sell medications that are contaminated, expired, too weak, too potent, or even counterfeit. Sites also may not warn you when a new medication could interact dangerously with drugs you already take. To protect yourself, never buy from a pharmacy that:

▸ does not require a prescription for prescription drugs.

▸ "prescribes" medicine based on an online form you fill out.

- does not offer a licensed pharmacist to answer your questions.

- does not provide a United States address and phone number to contact if problems occur.

- does not have the Digital Pharmacy accreditation (formerly VIPPS).

Digital Pharmacy accreditation means the pharmacy is licensed by the states where it operates and has passed the National Association of Boards of Pharmacy (NABP) requirements for quality and security. For an updated list of accredited digital pharmacies, visit the NABP Web site at *nabp.pharmacy,* or call 847-391-4406.

Check the fine print. For safety and savings, follow these tips before you order.

- Read the privacy policy. Make sure your financial and personal information won't be sold to others.

- Read the refund policy.

- Figure out how much your taxes and fees will cost. Sometimes they're more than your savings.

- Check whether the site promises that its security software encrypts and protects your information from hackers.

Reap big savings when you dare to compare. Keep practicing online safety so you can take advantage of opportunities like these to save a boatload on prescription drugs from now on. These price comparison tools help you find the best deals at local pharmacies and give you access to coupons. Here's how much they claim to help you save.

- RxSaver. Go to *rxsaver.com* and save up to 85 percent on your prescriptions.

- GoodRx. At *goodrx.com*, you could save up to 80 percent on brand name and generic drugs.

- Blink Health. Savings average about 60 percent at *blinkhealth.com* and, in some cases, can be 80 percent or more.

Gingivitis

Take the bite out of gum disease

Here's good news for your teeth. Unlike previous generations, the majority of baby boomers are expected to keep their own teeth for their whole lives, thanks to widespread water fluoridation, fluoride toothpastes, and improved dental care.

But not all is rosy in those tooth-filled mouths. About four in 10 adults aged 30 or older have gingivitis, or inflammation of the gums, which causes redness, swelling, pain, and bleeding when you brush your teeth. Gingivitis can lead to more serious gum disease called periodontitis. This could mean loss of connective tissue and bone that supports your teeth. Gum disease can also contribute to serious illnesses, like heart disease, stroke, diabetes, and pneumonia.

With a few inexpensive tools, attention to diet, and regular professional care, you can reverse the course of gum disease and avoid costly health problems.

3 simple ways to reduce your risk

Some people might be naturally prone to excess bacteria and plaque buildup on their gums, which leads to gum disease. Yet, certain things can make it worse — like diabetes, rheumatoid arthritis, and obesity; smoking or chewing tobacco; certain medications; poorly fitting bridgework or dentures; and menopause.

Not surprisingly, the greatest cause of gingivitis is not taking care of your teeth and gums. Follow these recommendations from the American Dental Association (ADA) to keep plaque-causing bacteria at bay.

▸ **Brush your teeth at least twice each day.** Do this carefully and thoroughly for at least two minutes using a soft-bristled brush that fits your mouth. Gently brush your tongue, too. Bacteria like to lurk there. Use toothpaste with fluoride that has the ADA seal of acceptance on the label.

▸ **Floss every day.** Yes, floss. Although only about 32 percent of American households actually use floss on a regular basis, dentists say it is the best — and simplest — way to remove plaque and food in tight spaces between teeth. You may have heard using mouthwash is as good as flossing. Many professionals say it can help in the fight against plaque, but so far, there's not enough evidence to prove it's a substitute for flossing.

▸ **Visit your dentist twice a year.** It's important to catch trouble quickly. Because early gingivitis may have few symptoms, you might not even know you have a problem until your dentist tells you.

By testing your saliva for certain bacteria, doctors can tell if you have mouth cancer even before you have symptoms. Saliva tests also check for periodontitis and other conditions.

Don't think you are off the hook when it comes to oral care if you wear partial or full dentures. Brush your dentures twice a day with a soft brush and a nonabrasive denture cleaner. Remove your dentures at night to soak, and clean your gums with a soft, wet cloth or soft toothbrush. Finally, visit your dentist regularly so he can check for signs of gum disease and mouth cancer.

Action plan for healthy gums

Likely your mother told you to stay away from sugar so your teeth wouldn't rot, but that's only part of the story. A study at Case Western Reserve University found that those who followed the USDA Food Pyramid recommendations lowered their risk of gum disease by 40 percent. USDA guidelines are different for each person based on age, weight, sex, and activity level, but in general they include:

▸ Lots of fruits, vegetables, whole grains, and low-fat dairy products. Research finds that eating three servings of whole grains every day can reduce your risk of gum disease.

▸ Plenty of lean meats, fish, poultry, eggs, beans, and nuts.

▸ Very little salt, sugar, trans fatty acids, and saturated fats. Trans fatty acids are found in hydrogenated oils, like margarine and vegetable shortening. Cheese, whole milk, fatty meat, and butter are high in saturated fats.

Besides this basic plan for good gum health, certain nutrients and foods can help protect you from gum disease.

Save money on dental care

You can save money on professional dental care without cutting back on visits. Dental schools offer low-cost treatment done by dental students who are closely supervised by licensed dentists. Or you can look for a clinical trial that needs people to test a new treatment. You might gain free or reduced-price care and even be paid for participating. Find a list of dental schools at *asdanet.org*. Click on "Get Into Dental School" then select "U.S. Dental Schools."

Energy or sports drinks, cola and non-cola soft drinks, and commercial lemonade can cause your tooth enamel to erode. If you drink these beverages, rinse out your mouth with water when finished.

Vitamin C. This famous vitamin is in charge of making collagen, which helps hold together your body's cells and tissues. It also supports your bones and teeth. Citrus fruits and juice, strawberries, sweet red peppers, and broccoli are good sources.

Vitamin D. Recent studies found its anti-inflammatory abilities might help gums heal faster and bleed less during dental exams. You can get vitamin D from fortified milk and fatty fish, like salmon and mackerel. When you're exposed to sunlight, your body makes vitamin D. Go outside and soak up some sunshine for about 15 minutes every day.

Polyphenols. These potent antioxidants, found in foods like cranberries, red grapes, blueberries, grape juice, and strawberries, seem to work by cleaning up the waste products of the body's immune system. That allows your immune system cells to attack more of the bacteria that cause gum disease.

Raisins. If you've always believed nature's candy is bad for your teeth, think again. Scientists have found that certain compounds in raisins, especially oleanolic acid, actually help kill the bacteria that cause gum disease and cavities. It also prevents bacteria from sticking to your teeth and forming plaque.

Garlic. An extract of this potent herb kills the bacteria that cause gingivitis. In a four-month clinical trial, aged garlic extract reduced inflammation and bleeding in participants' gums compared to a placebo group.

Your dentist can save your life

The best reason to take care of your teeth is to keep your beautiful white smile, right? Not quite. A recent survey found that nearly all doctors and dentists see a link between gum disease and other serious diseases. Taking good care of your teeth and gums might help ward off these life-threatening conditions:

▸ **Heart disease.** In one study, 91 percent of people with heart disease also suffered from serious gum disease. One theory is the same disease-causing bacteria that camp out in your mouth move through your bloodstream, eventually forming plaques in your arteries. Yet another idea is that inflammation caused by serious gum disease damages your blood vessel walls.

▸ **Stroke.** Severe gum disease can raise your risk of stroke by causing plaques to form in your carotid arteries, which supply blood to your brain. Reduced blood flow to the brain caused by a blockage can lead to a stroke.

▸ **Diabetes.** What comes first — diabetes or gum disease? Both these conditions can make the other worse. People with diabetes often experience dry mouth, which allows bacteria to build up and worsen gingivitis. Wounds, including small mouth infections, are also slower to heal for people with diabetes. On the other hand, some mouth infections can make it difficult to control blood sugar.

Sweet solution for unruly plaque

Xylitol, a natural sugar from fruits and other plants, has been shown in more than 300 studies to prevent tooth decay. This amazing sweetener works by blocking plaque-forming bacteria from sticking to the surface of teeth and gums. No plaque — no decay. It's now available in chewing gum, candy, and even toothpaste. Look for products containing xylitol as the only sweetener.

▸ **Runaway infections.** While it's not pleasant to imagine, an untreated infection in your mouth can spread to your bones, muscles, skin, heart — and even your brain. The result can be agonizing pain, severe inflammation, and even death in rare cases. So much for toughing out a toothache.

Broadband light, used to whiten teeth in your dentist's office, can be used to control gum disease. Research shows these lights quickly kill the most harmful strains of gingivitis-causing bacteria.

Not horrified yet? Gum disease may also be connected to pneumonia and mouth cancer. And don't forget the basic purpose of teeth — to help you eat a wide variety of foods. Studies have shown that people who keep more of their own teeth throughout life enjoy better nutrition as they age. Poor oral health can be very costly.

Give high-tech claims the brush-off

Just because it's newer doesn't mean it's better. That's important to remember when shopping for oral-care products. You may be tempted to spend more money on fancy toothbrushes, gadgets that sterilize, and toothpastes and mouthwashes that make big promises. Some features of these new products might be nice to have, but few are necessary to give you a cleaner mouth.

Pick the perfect toothbrush. You can pay as much as $140 for a rechargeable electric toothbrush. Those with timers can let you know when to stop brushing, and some with lights can alert you if you are pressing too hard on your gums. But as far as cleaning goes, in the right hands, the good old $2 variety does as good a job as any. The only exception might be brushes with circular movement in both directions, called rotation oscillation action, which do a better job of removing plaque from tight spaces.

Stay away from sterilizers. You like things clean, especially things you put in your mouth. That's why marketers have been successful with new devices made to sterilize your toothbrush. These gadgets, selling for as much as $100, use ultraviolet light to kill germs.

Remember, your mouth is already full of germs — around 700 kinds of microbes — most of which are harmless. Only certain types can lead to gingivitis when they remain in large numbers on your gums.

To keep your toothbrush clean, rinse it after use and let it air dry. If you have a lowered immune system or are getting over an infection, buy a new toothbrush more frequently than the usual recommendation of every three months.

Add this gum-friendly plant to your nightly routine

Ever heard of neem? It's a tree native to India and nearby countries, where it's been used to treat almost every condition under the sun — including gingivitis.

Neem twigs are often used in India as a sort of toothbrush, called a chewing stick. But neem has also been made into other products you're more familiar with. In one study, participants who used neem-based toothpaste had significantly less severe plaque and gingivitis than those who used conventional toothpaste.

Likely at work is neem's main active component, azadirachtin, which is antimicrobial. It attacks and breaks down bacterial cell walls, killing the threat and stopping the spread of bacteria.

If you're ready for a new way to protect against gingivitis, you can easily purchase neem toothpaste and mouthwash online from places like Wal-Mart, Walgreens, and Amazon.

Gout

Don't pay royally to treat the "disease of kings"

Gouch! If you are among the more than 9 million Americans who suffer from this form of arthritis, you understand how painful an attack can be. Uric acid crystals build up in the joints, often in the toes or fingers, causing sudden and severe pain, inflammation, and even fever.

Although you may think of gout as a men's disease, women suffer, too. It's true that men are struck with gout during mid-life twice as often as women, but that changes with age. After menopause, women's uric acid levels increase, putting them at greater risk for symptoms. Gout is equally common among men and women age 60 and older. Unlike men, who tend to have pain in a single toe, older women most often suffer from gout in several finger joints, which can become swollen and deformed.

The number of Americans with gout appears to be increasing, but there are some changes you can make to live with this "disease of kings" without paying royally.

Eat right and spend less on medicine

If you suffer from gout, you know it's caused by too much uric acid in the blood, sometimes brought on by eating foods rich in purines.

While it's nearly impossible to avoid all purines in food, you should steer clear of these troublemakers:

- red meats, including beef, pork, and lamb
- organ meats, like beef or pork liver
- some seafoods, such as anchovies, sardines, and herring
- chocolate, which can raise blood uric acid levels
- alcohol, including beer and wine

Some vegetables, like spinach and pinto beans, also contain lots of purines, but these don't seem to cause problems for people with gout. What's more, research has shown that some dietary choices can help you avoid a bout of gout.

- Dairy products, especially low-fat choices like skim milk and low-fat yogurt, seem to keep the amount of uric acid circulating in your blood under control.

Surprising causes of gout

Gout is not all about what you eat. Family history can determine whether your love of bacon will bring on a bout of pain, since some 20 percent of people with gout have a family history of the disease. Gout can also be brought on by some common medical treatments.

- thiazide diuretics, which are water pills taken to lower high blood pressure
- large doses of niacin, also called vitamin B3, sometimes prescribed for high cholesterol
- kidney, heart, or liver transplant

- Coffee helped lower uric acid levels in a recent study of 1,955 people ages 18 to 65.

- Cherries have long been known to lessen joint pain and the inflammation of gout and other types of arthritis. Although in a recent study, researchers had women eat a bowl of 45 cherries to test the effect, you can opt for dried cherries or cherry juice for relief.

- Water — your mother's good ol' standby advice actually works. Drinking lots of water can help flush out the extra uric acid that might be lurking, waiting to cause you more pain.

Ditch low-carb diet to cut your risk

It's no coincidence that the rate of obesity is rising at the same time as the number of gout cases. Boston researcher Dr. Hyon K. Choi found that men whose weight increased by more than 30 pounds after age 21 doubled their chances of getting gout.

A recent study showed that a natural chemical in onions — called quercetin — can lower uric acid levels. People in the study took quercetin supplements. But if you'd rather get it naturally, red onions provide the biggest bang for the buck. You'll need to eat about two-thirds of a red onion daily.

You better beware of low-carbohydrate diets, too. They might be all the rage, but they are not a good idea for people with gout. Because such plans have you eating lots of meat and other purine-rich food, while avoiding dairy products, they tend to raise uric acid levels. Stick to a healthy weight-loss plan involving moderate exercise and low-fat food choices. Don't go overboard — fasting can bring on a gout flare-up.

DASH your risk for painful attacks with this heart-smart plan

New research suggests that sticking to a heart-healthy meal plan — the Dietary Approaches to Stop Hypertension (DASH) diet — may lower your risk of gout.

That's according to a large study led by researchers at Harvard Medical School. The team followed the eating habits of more than 44,000 men over a whopping 26 years. None of them had a history of gout at the start of the study.

> Vitamin C reduces uric acid levels in your blood. A daily intake of 500 milligrams (mg) of vitamin C is recommended by health experts to get its full effect.

The scientists scored the people in the study on how closely they followed the DASH diet's emphasis on fruits and vegetables, nuts, beans, whole grains, and low-fat dairy. They also rated how closely their food choices matched the typical Western diet, which is high in red and processed meats, french fries, sweets, and refined grains.

After accounting for known risk factors like age, body mass index, and high blood pressure, the scientists found that higher DASH scores were tied to a lower risk of gout, whereas higher Western-diet scores were linked to a higher risk.

Unfortunately, the scientists weren't able to prove cause and effect. But, they say, the DASH diet may be a good all-around approach because it also treats high blood pressure — a condition that affects the majority of gout patients.

Tools easy on your joints and wallet

You can continue to enjoy your favorite hobbies even if gout has attacked your hands. Shop around for some of the many adaptive tools and aids designed for people who need a little help. The Arthritis Foundation picks some of the best to receive the Ease-of-Use commendation.

If your favorite hobby involves gardening or needlework, you can make smart choices and modify some of the tools you already have to keep your condition from draining your wallet.

Get a grip on gardening. If you like spending time in the dirt, try these tricks to work around your gout.

▶ Make time in the garden count. Decide which tasks are needed, and which you enjoy most, and delegate or skip the rest.

▶ Wear large, well-padded gloves to save your hands.

▶ Tape tool handles for less stress on your hands. Use electrical tape, foam padding, or Bubble Wrap for a better grip and extra cushioning.

▶ Try seed tape. Laying out a line of tape is easier than digging individual holes for seeds.

Keep your knack for needlework. Modifying or purchasing certain tools can help you continue to enjoy sewing and needlework.

▶ Use layers of tape or foam hair curlers (dig out your old pink ones) to create a better grip on knitting needles or crochet hooks.

▶ Many styles of needle threaders, from the simple to the spectacular, can save both your eyesight and your fingers.

▶ Switch from hand sewing to using your sewing machine whenever possible and you can save your fingers for those important projects where your beautiful stitches will be noticed.

▶ Fusible webbing, iron-on shapes, and fabric glue can help you avoid tedious and painful hand sewing. And the effect can be fantastic.

▶ The right scissors or rotary cutter can make a big difference in reducing hand stress. Try one of the new styles of spring-action or electric scissors, which keep your fingers from having to squeeze too hard.

Know your treatment options

Relieving pain and swelling is likely your top priority during a gout attack. Doctors have a few choices when it comes to prescribing drugs, depending on whether your body produces too much uric acid or simply can't get rid of it all. These drugs work, but some people suffer from serious side effects.

Steroid injections to the joint can help, too. The relief may last for only a few months, but steroids can be a good option if you can't take other pain medicines.

> Stay in bed during a gout flare-up and for at least 24 hours after, doctors advise, since movement can cause inflammation and yet another attack.

Pain relievers like naproxen (Aleve) and indomethacin (Indocin) can get you through a serious attack. These and other types of nonsteroidal anti-inflammatory drugs (NSAIDs) work well in people with no liver or kidney problems. But don't take aspirin for gout. In low doses, like the 81-milligram baby aspirin you take for your heart, it can actually bring on a gout attack.

Hair loss

Attack the problem at its roots

"Hair" today, gone tomorrow, right? For too many people, this phrase becomes more and more true as they age.

Roughly 50 percent of all men face the prospect of thinning or disappearing hair. Surprisingly, 75 percent of women older than 65 also experience some hair loss. Hair loss, or alopecia, is an age-old problem, and maybe that's why people stake their hopes — and their dollars — on outlandish claims and "magic" potions. Modern science has made progress, so you don't need to rely on empty promises.

If your head has been looking less like Rapunzel's and more like Kojak's, you can take steps now to slow or even reverse your hair loss. Some products and treatments are expensive, but in many cases you get what you pay for. Shop around and compare to find the best treatment for you.

Get top results with proven treatments

You finally admit you have a hair-loss problem, and now you want a solution. You can choose from all sorts of miraculous cures and "guaranteed" products, most with impressive test statistics and a convincing celebrity spokesperson. But if all these amazing cures work so well, why doesn't everyone enjoy a full head of hair?

The answer, of course, is that not all these promises are true. Researchers have tested a variety of products that claim to regrow hair or stop its loss, and a few have proven effective. Don't waste your money on the others.

Minoxidil (Rogaine) is a solution applied to the scalp. It's approved by the Food and Drug Administration (FDA) to treat pattern baldness. Scientists are not sure how minoxidil works, but it seems to stimulate inactive hair follicles to regrow hair and keep hair from falling out. If you stop using minoxidil, hair loss will continue. Side effects can include scalp irritation and some unwanted hair growth for women.

Finasteride (Propecia) is a pill approved by the FDA for men only. It works by blocking the conversion of testosterone to a byproduct (DHT) that damages hair follicles, so men may have some sexual side effects. Finasteride is not approved for women because of the chance for birth defects.

Certain drugs, like chemotherapy for cancer treatment, colchicine for gout, beta blockers, or anti-coagulants, can cause hair thinning or complete loss.

This treatment can slow hair loss and regrow hair, but these symptoms will come back if you stop taking it.

Hair transplantation is a permanent way to put hair back once it's gone. Available since 1952, hair transplants have greatly improved as they have become more common, with more than 80,000 Americans undergoing the treatment in one year. Unfortunately, the process won't work if you're completely bald because you must have areas of growing hair the surgeon can retrieve as donor follicles.

Help your hair from the inside out

A healthy crop of hair can be a sign of health and good nutrition. The reverse may also be true. Thinning hair may be related to what is missing from your diet. Long before drugs were developed to treat hair loss, people found natural remedies to help save their locks. But before you buy, consider the pros and cons of these supplements touted for hair loss.

Iron. For some cases of hair loss, low iron in the blood could make the problem worse. Even if your iron level is not low enough to signal anemia, it could be low enough to keep you from growing a thick crop of hair.

Not everyone agrees. But researchers at the Cleveland Clinic who study people with thinning hair check blood levels of ferritin — a protein that helps the body store iron — to see who's at risk. They have found that even when ferritin levels are in a range considered normal, many people still suffer from hair loss. The researchers think this is because growing hair follicles need more iron than other cells in the body. When they add iron supplements to other treatments, it seems to improve people's ability to grow hair.

But don't take iron supplements on your own. Talk to your doctor first, and ask him to check your ferritin level. Getting too much iron can be dangerous since your body can't easily get rid of the extra. Also, iron pills can cause constipation and stomach upset. Your best bet is to get more iron from your diet by eating foods such as spinach, beans, tofu, raisins, and lean beef.

Speedy weight loss brings on hair loss. If your diet doesn't include enough protein, iron, vitamin D, and other nutrients, your hair may get thinner along with your waistline.

Saw palmetto. This ancient remedy for hair loss might actually do the trick. It's an herb that works like the drug finasteride. It keeps testosterone from changing to a byproduct (DHT) that damages hair follicles. In fact, one study found that 60 percent of the men who tried it saw improved hair growth. However, this study was small, and the men were also taking another supplement, so saw palmetto might not be entirely responsible for the benefits. More research still needs to be done.

> It's normal to lose about 100–150 hairs each day as your locks progress through the normal cycle of growing, resting, shedding, and regrowth.

Fenugreek. Long used as a spice, this legume has been studied to see if it can lower blood sugar in people with diabetes, fight stomach ulcers, and battle colon cancer. Some people believe it may also slow hair loss and help with regrowth, but little scientific evidence has shown this effect.

A Danish product called Folligro is a fenugreek combination packaged especially for people who battle hair loss. You may want to think twice about herbal remedies with fenugreek until more research is done. And avoid fenugreek completely if you regularly take nonsteroidal anti-inflammatory drugs (NSAIDs) because the combination can cause bleeding.

Hair cloning: hope for the future

It may seem farfetched, but researchers are working on ways of multiplying, or "cloning," a person's hair follicle cells. If this method of regrowing hair works, you would have a few follicle cells removed, let them multiply in a lab dish, then have them "planted" where you need them. Because hair cells appear to adapt to changes in location and will even grow on different people, this kind of regrowth is likely to be possible in a few years.

4 ways to make the most of what you have

You can spend a lot of money and effort trying to make your thinning hair grow back. Or you can look for other solutions. Here are four options to think about.

Consider a cut. If you wear your hair long and pulled into a ponytail or bun, you may show more exposed scalp than you need to. A shorter cut that allows bangs or layers of hair to cover any thinning spots can help make the most of your remaining hair.

Extend your look. Hair extensions are human or synthetic hair that is woven in, sewn on, or glued to your own hair. It can be a natural-looking way to improve your appearance. Styles and prices vary widely, but you can expect to spend upwards of $200–$2,500 for well-applied extensions of good-quality human hair. Extensions require maintenance every two to 12 weeks depending on whether they are glued or sewn in, adding to the cost. To save money, you can get do-it-yourself clip-in extensions, but you must remove them every night.

Pump up the volume. You've probably seen ads for shampoos, conditioners, and styling products designed to add volume to hair. These can help make your thinning mane appear thicker. In addition, certain products help camouflage thinning hair.

▸ Masking lotions are applied to the scalp and base of the hair to reduce the contrast between the two. They stay in place during swimming and styling but wash out with shampoo. Pick a lotion to match your hair color.

▸ Powders matched to your hair color can coat remaining hairs, allowing them to spread out for better scalp coverage. These last through exercise and the swimming pool, but they come out when you wash your hair.

▸ Products containing microfibers of keratin, the same protein that makes up hair and nails, are shaken over the thinning area to bond with the hair. Manufacturers promise their products will last through bad weather but not a dip in the swimming pool.

Cover up the problem. Wigs have come a long way in the past few years. Nowadays they are realistic-looking and comfortable and won't fall off if you put them on correctly. A wig stylist can help you select one to match your hairstyle and color if you show her an old photograph of yourself. Prices vary widely, from around $195 for synthetic hair to $1,500 for human hair. If that's more than you want to spend, make a fashion statement instead. Tie a scarf around your head, or wear a hat.

Vitamin E tackles hair loss head on

Can a common vitamin re-grow thinning hair? This study suggests it.

Volunteers with significant hair loss took a supplement of tocotrienol — a form of vitamin E — for eight months during this trial from the University of Science Malaysia. All of the volunteers had experienced hair loss for two to five years prior to the study. Those who took 100 milligrams of tocotrienol daily grew more hair than those who took a placebo.

More research needs to be done, so talk with your doctor before taking a vitamin E supplement for hair loss.

Calm your nerves to save your locks

It's a vicious cycle. Stressful events or lifestyles can lead to loss of hair, and hair loss can trigger extra stress. Many people — both men and women — seem overly bothered by the idea their hair is thinning.

But hair has symbolic value far beyond the protection and warmth it provides for the head. It can be a symbol of beauty for women and a sign of youth for men. Losing it can be traumatic, and studies have found that people experiencing hair loss can feel depressed, ashamed, angry, and embarrassed. Unfortunately, certain hair-loss conditions are made even worse by these stressful attitudes.

Poor choice of hairstyles — excess use of hot combs or tightly pulled braids, pony-tails, or topknots — can lead to temporary or even permanent loss of hair.

To stop this vicious cycle, doctors recommend a variety of stress-reduction techniques, such as exercise, music, massage, and relaxation. Use these tricks to help yourself feel better while your hair is thinning. You'll find details in the *Depression* chapter in *Top tips for beating the blues*.

A laser light could rouse your scalp

Shock your follicles back into growth mode with a treatment straight out of the Jetsons. It's called low-level laser therapy (LLLT), and it was given the nod of approval by the FDA in 2011.

Caps, headbands, helmets, combs — these are all pricey devices that promise lush tresses through laser treatments. But can they really wake up your lethargic locks?

Proponents of LLLT say yes. While LLLT doesn't promise to bring dead follicles back to life, it can stimulate those that have slowed down production, so you see thicker, fuller hair.

Studies have shown — and satisfied customers report — that LLLT is a safe and effective treatment for androgenetic and chemotherapy-induced alopecia, as well as alopecia areata. George Jetson would be pleased.

Dollars&Sense
Foreign drugs — are they worth the risks?

Americans spend more money buying drugs than do people in other countries — an average of $1,011 per person in 2014 compared to $669 in Canada and $497 in the United Kingdom. One reason is many brand-name drugs cost more in the United States because the government does not regulate prices.

You've probably heard of people buying drugs in other countries, either by traveling to Canada, Mexico, or overseas — or by ordering them online. Saving money may be tempting, but there are a few things you should consider.

Examine the facts. Before you hop on the next plane, you need to think about other factors like where the prescriptions are coming from and what the rules are. Evaluate these points to see if buying foreign meds is the right choice for you.

▸ Cost. Factor in the expenses from shipping, travel, and currency conversion and then compare the prices to U.S. generics. You might find you won't save any money.

▸ Safety. Foreign tests and guidelines don't always meet the standards set by the U.S. Food and Drug Administration (FDA). Talk to a doctor you trust to avoid buying unsafe medicine.

▸ Legality. Importing unapproved prescriptions is illegal, but the FDA makes certain exceptions. For example, if you have a serious condition and the drug you need is not available in the U.S., they may allow you to bring in a 90-day supply. Make sure you meet all the criteria before taking the plunge.

Understand what you're buying. Don't assume your prescription carries the same name in another country as it does at home. The Institute for Safe Medication Practices issued a safety alert in 2015 about drugs sold in other countries that have different ingredients as U.S. drugs with the same names. You may pop into a drugstore while on vacation in Europe or South America to buy Flomax only to get a different drug with different effects.

Be a smart shopper. If you've compared prices and still think buying drugs from a foreign pharmacy is your ticket to savings, take these precautions to stay safe and avoid scams.

- Go in person. If you can travel to a brick-and-mortar drugstore, you can be more certain of getting the drug you think you're getting. You can also talk to the pharmacist about your drugs, side effects, and possible interactions.

- Choose an Internet or mail-order pharmacy carefully. Be sure it has a working toll-free phone number answered by live operators, is located at a physical street address, and requires a prescription for your drug.

- Get information at *www.pharmacychecker.com*. You can compare prices and get ratings on online pharmacies.

- Sign up at *www.safemedicines.org* for warnings through the SafeMeds Alert System. Government alerts about counterfeit and bad drugs will be sent to your e-mail address. It's a free service.

- If you purchase over the Internet, double-check the Web site's security. To make sure your personal information will be kept safe on any Web site, look carefully at the site's URL. Does it begin with "https" instead of just "http"? The "s" at the end stands for "secure." A good sign. It means your info is being encrypted.

  Next, look for the lock icon somewhere in your web browser's window. But don't assume the lock means the site is secure. Click on it and read the Web site's security and authenticity. That will help give you some peace of mind when doing business online.

Heart disease

Bypass high costs of standard treatments

Heart disease is the world's No. 1 killer — so preventing heart disease should be your No. 1 priority. When you have heart disease, your coronary arteries, the blood vessels around your heart, become clogged or blocked. This can lead to serious problems, including heart attack, angina or chest pain, heart failure, and an irregular heartbeat called arrhythmia.

Lifestyle changes, such as a healthy diet and regular exercise, can help prevent heart disease. But you may also need medication. New drugs promise greater protection than ever, but at what cost?

Find out what steps you can take to guard against heart disease, and how you can help your heart without hurting your pocketbook.

Little pill has big benefits — and hazards

Popping a daily aspirin is an easy, cheap, and effective way to ward off a heart attack or stroke. It works as a blood thinner so it gives your body its own natural, clot-busting protection. But aspirin works differently for men and women. And it's not recommended for everyone.

Recent studies show that daily aspirin therapy helps men prevent heart attacks and women prevent strokes, but not vice versa. Another large study found that aspirin might help prevent heart attacks in women over age 65. Younger women, perhaps because of the protection of estrogen, did not benefit from aspirin.

Your doctor may recommend aspirin if you're at risk for heart disease or if you've already had a heart attack. In fact, researchers recently discovered that taking aspirin before and after bypass surgery could save 8,000 lives a year in the United States.

> Air pollution, loud noise, and high humidity can harm your heart. If you can get away, head for the mountains and take an uphill walk. It's good for your heart.

But if you're perfectly healthy, you may be doing more harm than good. Because aspirin works as a blood thinner to keep your blood from clumping and clotting, it boosts your risk for major bleeding and even hemorrhagic stroke. Other possible problems include ulcers and kidney failure.

Remember, aspirin can interact with other drugs. Let your doctor know which medications, including vitamins, supplements, and herbs, you are taking. If your doctor recommends aspirin therapy, follow his instructions carefully.

'Shocking' way to save your life

You don't always have time to call "911" when you experience signs of a heart attack. Some heart attacks, called sudden cardiac arrest, stop your heart right away.

For cases like that, consider buying a home defibrillator. These devices use an electric shock to restart a heart attack victim's heart. They come with instructions and are easy to use, but it's a good idea to get some training. You can never be too prepared for an emergency.

There's just one problem — you can't use a defibrillator on yourself. So if you live alone, it doesn't make much sense to buy one. But if you live with family or your family spends a lot of time at your house, a home defibrillator can be a lifesaver.

2 vaccines that could save your heart

Need another reason to get your vaccinations? Here are two.

- A flu shot could slash your risk of a heart attack, stroke, or heart failure within the next year — by a third if you have a history of heart disease and by as much as 50 percent if you've had a recent heart attack. Experts aren't completely sure how the vaccine protects you, but they think it may trigger your immune system to produce heart-defending proteins.

- Get the pneumonia vaccine and you protect your heart against tiny lesions caused by the *Streptococcus pneumoniae* bacteria. According to Carlos Orihuela, associate professor of microbiology and immunology at the University of Texas Health Science Center, a case of severe pneumonia could leave your heart permanently scarred and possibly explain the link between this dangerous infection and heart failure.

Top questions to ask before heart surgery

Heart surgery, no matter how minor the procedure, is scary enough. But it's even scarier when you don't know where to have the surgery done. How do you know you're getting the best care?

Often, your local community hospital can provide great care and cost much less. It all comes down to experience — the more, the better. Ideally, you want a hospital that performs at least 450 bypass surgeries a year. The surgeon you choose should do 125 or more each year.

Feel free to ask your surgeon questions about his experience, including number of operations, death rates, and rates of other complications. A little research can go a long way toward finding the best care — and much-needed peace of mind.

5 ways to keep your heart healthy

You can't control all of your risk factors for heart disease. For instance, you can't change your age, gender, or family history. But you can do something about the others. Is it possible to lower blood pressure, cholesterol, and blood sugar without expensive drugs? The experts say yes.

In a 12-week study at the Center for Heart Disease Prevention in Savannah, Ga., people with risk factors such as high cholesterol or high blood pressure managed to lower these levels significantly by sticking to an individually tailored exercise plan, meal plan, and other lifestyle changes.

Making these changes takes some work, but it's cheaper than drugs — without any side effects. Eating a healthy diet, exercising regularly, losing weight if you're overweight, and quitting smoking will put you on the path to a healthy heart, but there are other steps you can take.

Cut your chances of a heart attack by 74 percent — without drugs, surgery, diet, or exercise. The secret? Learn how to handle mental stress, which can trigger a heart attack. People with heart disease drastically lowered their risk for heart attack with four months of stress management training.

Hostility, intense arguments, and road rage have all been linked to heart attacks. Finding a healthier, more productive way to deal with stress can mean the difference between life and death. Along with stress management, try these helpful tips for better heart health.

▸ **Laugh more.** Laughter relaxes blood vessels and increases blood flow. Rent a funny movie or spend time with humorous friends or relatives.

▸ **Skip the siesta.** Daily afternoon naps can boost your risk of a heart attack, according to a Costa Rican study.

▸ **See the glass as half full.** Optimism helps ward off heart disease. A Dutch study found that optimistic men were half as likely to die from cardiovascular disease, including heart attack, stroke, and coronary heart disease, as their less optimistic counterparts.

▸ **Listen to music.** Italian researchers found that music may have a beneficial relaxing effect on your heart.

▸ **Get a pet.** Studies have linked pet ownership to a reduced risk of heart disease.

Reap 'fin-tastic' protection from fish

Ever wish for an easy way to fight heart disease? Well, stop wishing and start fishing. Eating fish does wonders for your heart. That's because it's rich in omega-3 fatty acids. Researchers who recently examined several studies determined that eating fish lowers heart disease risk by roughly 10 percent and fatal heart disease risk by nearly 20 percent.

A recent Greek study found that eating fish reduces the risk for heart attacks or chest pain by 38 percent. Oddly, the benefits stopped at 5 ounces of fish a week. More fish did not mean increased benefits.

Fish oil helps heart attack survivors live longer, fights inflammation, lowers elevated heart rates, and even counteracts the damage that air pollution can do to your heart.

So why don't more people eat fish? Maybe because they're worried about pollutants. Reports of excessive mercury and contaminants called PCBs have called into question the safety of farm-raised fish, the kind most often available in supermarkets.

Brushing and flossing can save your heart, as well as your teeth. That's because the inflammation that comes with gum disease also boosts your risk for heart disease.

Don't let the fear of mercury and other toxins turn you into a landlubber. The proven heart benefits of eating fish far outweigh the slight risk of developing cancer from any contaminants. In fact, the American Heart Association still recommends you eat fatty fish twice a week.

But, just to be safe, you can take the following measures to limit mercury and PCB exposure.

▸ Avoid tilefish, shark, swordfish, and king mackerel.

▸ Choose fish lower in mercury. These include salmon, herring, sardines, shad, trout, mackerel, and whitefish.

▸ Pay attention to state advisories about the safety of fish caught in local lakes, rivers, and coastal areas.

▸ When cooking farm-raised salmon, grill or broil it to let the juices drip out, cook the fish until the internal temperature reaches 175 degrees Fahrenheit, and remove the skin before eating.

Some experts even recommend taking fish oil supplements rather than eating fish in order to avoid toxins. But supplements come with their own concerns. A recent study found that fish oil supplements might cause arrhythmia in some people.

Help your heart with a cup of coffee

Wake up and smell the coffee. Better yet, pour yourself a cup. A recent study found that drinking one to three cups of coffee a day might help protect you from heart disease. That's because coffee, rich in antioxidants, fights inflammation, which plays a major role in the development of heart disease. This stands in contrast to a previous study, which found that lifelong caffeine consumption might contribute to heart disease.

The type of coffee you drink may make a difference. Drinking filtered coffee does not appear to boost your risk of heart disease, even if you drink six cups or more a day. However, unfiltered or boiled coffee, such as the kind you make with a French press, may be harmful because it contains substances that raise cholesterol levels.

Coffee may also be dangerous if your body metabolizes it slowly. Because of an inherited trait, some people metabolize coffee slower than others. Unfortunately, this puts you at much greater risk for a heart attack. If coffee makes you feel weak or lightheaded, quickens your pulse, or causes pain in your chest, don't drink it.

Drinking coffee right before exercising may cause problems because it narrows your blood vessels, which decreases blood flow through the arteries supplying oxygen to your heart. If you start your day with a cup of coffee, wait at least an hour before exercising.

If coffee isn't your thing, drink tea instead. It's also chock-full of antioxidants and other health benefits.

Go nuts — boost blood flow to heal your heart

Lay all your blood vessels in a line, and you could circle the Earth four times. Veins, arteries, and capillaries cover a lot of ground. And to keep them working in tiptop shape, you need to make sure they stay healthy and flexible. Pistachios help you do that in two major ways.

Clear out buildup with a handful a day. Stockpiles of cholesterol block blood flow in your arteries, increasing your risk for heart problems. But pistachios could put a stop to all that, says a recent study published in *Nutrition*.

Lower blood pressure, heart disease, and diabetes and even reverse memory loss in seniors. Powerful nutrients in natural cocoa can do it all. But don't grab a glass of milk to wash down your dark chocolate treat. Milk can ruin the benefits by keeping antioxidants from being absorbed.

Researchers divided participants with raised cholesterol into two groups. For three months, both groups made healthy lifestyle changes, but only one got to eat pistachios.

Just one-third cup of these nutty treats a day bumped up good HDL cholesterol and lowered bad cholesterol. That means a healthy diet with good exercise habits — plus a handful of pistachios — can lead to healthier blood vessels.

Where does this protection come from? Antioxidants like lutein, beta carotene, and vitamin E.

Relieve pressure with the No. 1 nut. Nuts also take on high blood pressure. And pistachios are particularly qualified for the job.

A clever combo of healthy fats, phytosterols, and other nutrients work together to take the stress off your blood vessels, giving your heart a break.

A recent review of more than 20 studies, published in the *American Journal of Clinical Nutrition*, shows that eating pistachios lowers BP better than other nuts. Just don't undo the benefits by feasting on a bag of salted pistachios. Salt can hike up blood pressure without warning.

Ketchup's secret weapon battles high cholesterol

This saucy condiment is good for more than just flavoring your burger and fries. Research proves that lycopene, found naturally in tomatoes and tomato-based products like ketchup, may help lower your cholesterol naturally.

Lycopene is an antioxidant that wipes out free radicals before they can attach to cells and cause problems such as inflammation. When LDL cholesterol meets up with free radicals it becomes damaged — or oxidized — and eventually turns into plaque that clogs up your arteries.

One study showed that tomato juice, spaghetti sauce, and concentrated lycopene all helped double blood levels of lycopene and significantly lower oxidized LDL. And, amazingly, they did the job in just one week.

In analyzing more than 55 years of lycopene studies, scientists found this super antioxidant drops LDL levels by about 10 percent, similar to low doses of statin drugs. Study participants ate at least 25 milligrams of lycopene each day — the amount found in a cup of tomato juice or less than half a cup of spaghetti sauce.

Those foods are easy to add to your daily menu, and they're healthier than a ketchup-laden burger and fries. Here are some other ways to add lycopene to your meals.

▸ Breakfast — eat half a pink grapefruit.

▸ Lunch — enjoy a warm bowl of tomato soup.

▸ Dinner — dig into a hearty meal of pasta and marinara sauce. Or enjoy a low-cheese pizza with sun-dried tomatoes and plenty of sauce.

▸ Dessert — have a slice of watermelon.

High blood pressure
Smart ways to stop silent killer

High blood pressure can sneak up on you — and kill you. This serious condition, also known as hypertension, often has no symptoms. You may not know you have it until you get it checked at your doctor's office.

Blood pressure, which refers to the force of your blood as it moves through your blood vessels, is measured in millimeters of mercury, or mm Hg. It includes both systolic pressure, when your heart contracts, and diastolic pressure, when your heart relaxes between contractions. Systolic pressure comes first in a blood pressure reading. A reading of 140/90 or higher indicates high blood pressure. You want to keep your blood pressure below 120/80. Anything higher falls under the label "prehypertension," a risky condition recently recognized by health experts. Consider prehypertension a warning sign.

If left untreated, high blood pressure can lead to several serious health problems, including stroke, heart disease, heart failure, kidney disease, and blindness. Luckily, high blood pressure can be controlled with medication, as well as changes in diet and lifestyle.

10 terrific tips for reducing blood pressure

You can fight high blood pressure without risky drugs. Just follow these steps to lower blood pressure the natural way.

- Reduce salt. This means not only salt from your saltshaker but also the sodium in processed foods.

- Cut back on fat, red meat, and sweets — including sweetened drinks.

- Eat more fruits, vegetables, and whole grains.

- Maximize your minerals. Potassium, magnesium, and calcium play key roles in controlling your blood pressure, so make sure your diet provides them. It's as easy as reaching for beans and bananas. Beans are a good source of magnesium, while bananas are packed with potassium. To boost your calcium intake, try nonfat and low-fat dairy products.

- Limit alcohol. This means no more than two drinks a day for a man and one for a woman.

- Exercise regularly. Recent studies show that a 30-minute brisk walk each day can dramatically lower your blood pressure.

- Lose weight. As your weight decreases, so will your blood pressure.

- Quit smoking. It stiffens your arteries.

- Get enough sleep. Sleeping five hours or less a night may boost your risk of high blood pressure.

- Relax. Listen to music, get a massage, spend time with loved ones, or find other ways to reduce stress.

Sticking to these simple lifestyle and dietary changes can dramatically lower your blood pressure and help you avoid blood pressure medication entirely. That's what researchers discovered in the PREMIER study — 98 percent of those with high blood pressure became completely free of their medicine — with their doctor's approval — when they followed this simple advice.

The people in the study lost weight, exercised, reduced salt and alcohol intake, and followed the National Heart, Lung, and Blood Institute's Dietary Approaches to Stop Hypertension (DASH) diet — which stresses many of the dietary tips listed earlier. For more information about the DASH diet, you can download *Your Guide to Lowering Your Blood Pressure with DASH* by visiting the NHLBI Health Information Center online at *nhlbi.nih.gov/files/docs/public/ heart/new_dash.pdf.*

Drink up to drive blood pressure down

Pour yourself a glass of skim milk and you might skim your risk of developing high blood pressure in half. In a two-year study of nearly 6,000 people, those who had more than two or three daily servings of skim milk and other nonfat dairy products were half as likely to develop high blood pressure as people who rarely or never consumed these foods.

You can sip your way to lower blood pressure with the following beverages as well.

▸ **Grape juice.** In a Korean study, men drinking Concord grape juice significantly lowered both their systolic and diastolic blood pressure. Natural compounds called flavonoids found in grape juice likely deserve the credit.

▸ **Cocoa.** Drinking a special flavonol-rich cocoa beverage improved blood vessel function in healthy men and women in one small study. Look for this special flavonol-rich cocoa in CocoaVia products.

▸ **Fermented milk.** A Finnish study found that this popular Scandinavian beverage, made by adding the good bacteria *Lactobacillus* to milk, lowered blood pressure by about three points after 10 weeks. Fermented milk works in the same manner as ACE inhibitors, by blocking angiotensin-converting enzyme, a chemical that raises blood pressure.

If you need a cup of coffee to get going in the morning, here's some good news. Coffee boosts blood pressure in the short run, but regular coffee drinking does not seem to have an effect on

developing high blood pressure.
Yet, if you already have high
blood pressure, you may want to
limit your coffee consumption.
Other beverages that may raise
your blood pressure include
beer, wine, and colas — including diet colas.

Religion is not only good for
your soul, it's good for your
heart. Regular religious activity,
such as attending church and
praying, has been linked to
lower blood pressure.

One beverage you should
never drink if you're taking high
blood pressure medicine is
grapefruit juice. This fruit juice will drive your blood pressure to
toxic levels. That's because when you take calcium-channel blockers
with grapefruit juice, you end up with a much higher — and dangerous — amount of the drugs in your body. Chemicals in grapefruit
juice called furanocoumarins are responsible for this dangerous
interaction.

4 tasty ways to defeat the silent killer

What you eat has a big impact on your blood pressure. Perhaps the
best approach is to follow the DASH diet, which stresses eating
more fruits, vegetables, whole grains, and low-fat dairy products
while limiting salt, fat, alcohol, and sweets. But also make room for
the following foods, which just might give you an edge in the battle
against high blood pressure.

Celery. Long a staple of Chinese medicine, this crunchy vegetable
contains compounds called pthalides, which relax the muscles lining
your blood vessels. This allows them to dilate, or widen, so blood can
get through more easily. Four stalks of celery should do the trick.

Potatoes. Scientists discovered that potatoes contain
kukoamines, chemicals that lower blood pressure. Kukoamines
were previously only known to occur in an exotic plant used in
Chinese medicine. You'll preserve the health benefits of kukoamines
by boiling rather than frying your potatoes.

Fish. Several studies show that eating fish or taking fish oil supplements lowers blood pressure. The omega-3 fatty acids in fish help relax the cells lining your arteries, which improves circulation. Besides fatty fish like salmon, mackerel, or tuna, you can get omega-3 from flaxseed, canola oil, walnuts, wheat germ, and some green leafy vegetables, like collard and turnip greens.

Chocolate. A Dutch study found that older men who ate about a third of a bar of chocolate a day had lower blood pressure. Cocoa beans contain flavonols — natural compounds that can help keep your blood vessels working as they should.

Uncover hidden sources of salt

Salt, also known as sodium chloride, is an important mineral that is 40 percent sodium and 60 percent chloride. Unfortunately, sodium can wreak havoc with your blood pressure. Health experts recommend getting no more than 2,300 milligrams a day, but that's tough to do — especially when you don't know how much salt lurks in foods you eat every day.

The American Medical Association (AMA) says the best approach is to cut back on restaurant meals and limit how many processed foods you eat. When you prepare your own food, using fresh fruits, vegetables, skinless poultry and fish, nuts and legumes, and non-tropical vegetable oils, you can control how much salt you are getting.

Salt can also pop up in some surprising places, like your medication. Among over-the-counter drugs, antacids, laxatives, anti-inflammatory drugs, and cold medicines may contain large amounts of sodium. To find out how much sodium is hiding in the medication you take, read the labels on over-the-counter drugs. And ask your pharmacist to check the package inserts that come with prescription drugs.

And ask your pharmacist to check the package inserts that come with prescription drugs.

Steer clear of sodium hiding in your favorite foods

Watch out for these popular foods that contain more sodium than you might think.

Food	Serving size	Amount of sodium
frozen buttermilk pancakes	3 pancakes	815 mg
jarred spaghetti sauce	1/2 cup	525 mg
canned chicken noodle soup	1 cup	474 mg
low-fat cottage cheese	1/2 cup	459 mg
canned mushrooms	1/2 cup	331 mg
kosher dill pickles	1 spear	306 mg
unfrosted chocolate cake	1 slice	299 mg
light Italian salad dressing	2 tbsp	228 mg
rye bread	1 slice	211 mg
ketchup	1 tbsp	167 mg

Walk your way to healthier blood pressure

Get off the couch and start moving if you want to lower your blood pressure. Aim for at least 30 minutes of moderate exercise, such as walking, cycling, or swimming, most days of the week. Studies show regular exercise can shave three or four points off your blood pressure reading.

Blood pressure tends to shoot up in cold weather and go down in hot weather. However, an Italian study found that in people over age 65 nighttime blood pressure actually increased in hot weather.

If you already have high blood pressure, you may be reluctant to exercise because of the temporary rise in blood pressure that comes with activity. Experts say that it is safe for older people with mild high blood pressure to work out. Just check with your doctor before beginning any exercise program.

Sure, it's safe, you might say, but who has time to exercise? You do, as long as you can spare 10 minutes now and then. An Indiana University study found that four 10-minute sessions on a treadmill lowered blood pressure just as much as one continuous 40-minute session — and the effects lasted longer. So if you don't have time for a long walk, try squeezing in three or four short ones during your day.

Every little movement helps. You don't need to come up with an elaborate exercise routine or pay big bucks to join a gym. Just performing everyday activities, like gardening or walking up and down stairs, can help. A seven-year Japanese study of middle-age men found that those who were the most active in everyday life were much less likely to develop high blood pressure.

To see how many calories you can burn just by doing household chores or running errands, check out the chart in the *Gallstones* chapter.

High blood pressure linked to insomnia

You may not be too worried about your sleepless nights. After all, if you're tired during the day, you can take naps to catch up. But beware of sleeping too little during the night — you may see your blood pressure jump as a result.

When you sleep, your body relaxes, your heart slows down, and your blood pressure drops. But if you only sleep for short periods at a time, your blood pressure may stay elevated. A study showed that sleeping five hours or less a night could boost your risk for this dangerous condition.

If you suffer from insomnia, don't delay getting treatment. It's one condition that affects all aspects of your health.

Short-circuit dangerous drug interactions

Even if you eat right and exercise, sometimes you need medication to keep your blood pressure under control. But many blood pressure drugs come with important warnings. Here are a few to watch out for.

Nix nifedipine. Lowering your blood pressure with short-acting nifedipine, a calcium channel blocker, can cause a heart attack. High doses of this common medicine used to treat high blood pressure are especially dangerous. Your doctor may not think to tell you about this, so make sure to ask about safer alternatives.

Pay attention to potassium. ACE inhibitors can boost the level of potassium in your blood. Potassium can be good for your heart, but too much in your blood can be fatal — and this high blood pressure medicine can make it skyrocket. Use caution when taking ACE inhibitors, especially if you're also taking potassium supplements or potassium-sparing diuretics (water pills).

Pass on painkillers. Pain pills and some blood pressure drugs do not mix. Nonsteroidal anti-inflammatory drugs (NSAIDs), such as ibuprofen, may blunt the effectiveness of ACE inhibitors. They may also raise your blood pressure.

Dodge diabetes. While some drugs help control your blood pressure, they may increase your risk for other conditions — like diabetes. Common prescription drugs that may actually cause type 2 diabetes include diuretics and beta blockers. What's more, they might also boost your stroke risk. Are you unknowingly taking them? Ask your doctor if other options would be safer. Keep in mind that the benefits of these drugs may outweigh the risks. Never stop taking a drug your doctor prescribed without his approval.

Check your BP like a pro

For many people, the intimidating atmosphere of a doctor's office results in higher blood pressure readings. This phenomenon is called "white coat hypertension."

To make sure your doctor's presence is not affecting your blood pressure reading, consider buying a home monitor. Do-it-yourself monitoring may be more convenient, less costly, and even more accurate than standard approaches. It also makes you more likely to keep your blood pressure under control.

A Finnish study found that using a home device works just as well as ambulatory monitoring, which involves wearing a monitor that automatically records your blood pressure over a 24-hour period.

You can buy an aneroid monitor, which comes with a cuff, bulb, dial gauge, and stethoscope, for $20 to $40. If you have hearing or vision problems or arthritis, this manually operated monitor may be difficult for you to use.

Electronic monitors, which range from $30 to $125, come with a cuff that automatically inflates or deflates and a digital screen, making them easier to use. Choose an arm monitor rather than a wrist or fingertip model for a more accurate reading.

No matter which device you use, follow these tips for accurately measuring your blood pressure at home.

▶ Do not smoke or have any caffeine in the 30 minutes before you take your blood pressure.

▶ Sit and rest for 5 minutes before you begin.

▶ Average the results of two or more readings, taken at least a minute apart, to determine your blood pressure.

Remember to get your blood pressure checked by a doctor at least once a year, even if you are monitoring it yourself at home.

Up to half of those with sleep apnea also have high blood pressure. Luckily, a technique called continuous positive airway pressure (CPAP), which delivers air through a mask while you sleep, helps both conditions.

Tame tension to heal your heart

Some people think the word hypertension means you have too much stress. But it actually has nothing to do with emotional stress. Tension refers to the physical pressure of blood against your artery walls— and hyper means it's way too high.

Maybe this confusion is why less than half of people with high blood pressure have it under control. Lowering blood pressure takes more than just managing your stress levels. That said, adding stress-lowering strategies to your daily routine may be a helpful addition to your other treatments. Try these research-supported ways for relaxing.

Tune in to the classics. Want to rewind high blood pressure? Lay back and listen to Mozart's Symphony No. 40 in G minor. Classical music lowers your blood pressure better than upbeat pop songs like the works of ABBA, a study found. "Dancing Queen" is great for having a ball, but if you want to relax, sit with the symphonies for about 25 minutes.

Bring back an ancient practice. Tai Chi, a gentle, graceful form of exercise, is great for all ages. This Chinese tradition gets its heart-healing powers from fluid movements that focus on posture, coordination, and breathing patterns. One study showed it lowered systolic blood pressure by more than nine points.

Simmer down. By watching married couples have tense conversations for just 15 minutes, researchers could predict who would have health problems more than 20 years later. Are you a hothead? You may be setting yourself up for high blood pressure. Before you lose your temper, take a few deep breaths and calm yourself down.

Get a grip: Simple way to squeeze out high blood pressure

Want to add a boost to your exercise routine? Crush high blood pressure with isometric hand grippers.

It's unsurprising that experts give grippers two thumbs up. They were first studied in the 60s, when scientists noticed a trend. Fighter pilots training with hand-grip exercises to keep from blacking out during turns and dives had lower blood pressure.

A recent study showed that hand-grip exercises helped drop systolic blood pressure 10 points and diastolic pressure five points over 10 weeks.

You can easily find hand grippers online or at your local sporting goods store and try them yourself. Just squeeze for three minutes and rest five minutes. Repeat five times. Do this three days a week, and you'll be on your way to better blood pressure.

High cholesterol

Win the war with simple, low-cost tactics

Your body needs cholesterol to function, but you can have too much of a good thing. When you have high cholesterol, you put yourself at risk for atherosclerosis, heart disease, heart attack, and stroke. You may even increase your risk for Alzheimer's disease.

Cholesterol comes in two main forms. LDL, also called "bad" cholesterol, carries cholesterol to your artery walls. HDL, known as "good" cholesterol, whisks cholesterol to your liver and out of your body. You want to lower your LDL levels while boosting your levels of HDL.

Everyone should strive for LDL levels below 160 mg/dL and HDL levels above 40 mg/dL. But new guidelines call for even lower LDL for those at greater risk for heart attack. People at moderate risk should aim for 130 mg/dL or lower, while those at higher risk should shoot for 100 mg/dL or lower. People at the greatest risk should set a goal of less than 70 mg/dL. Your doctor will help you determine your ideal cholesterol goals.

Healthy habits hammer high cholesterol

Watch television or open a magazine, and you'll see plenty of advertisements for the latest cholesterol-lowering drugs. You might think popping pills is the only way to control your cholesterol. But eating right and making simple lifestyle changes can work just as well as drugs — and may even help you avoid them entirely.

It all starts with your diet. Some foods, like eggs, contain cholesterol, but saturated fats, the kind found in meat and dairy products, raise your cholesterol level more than anything else in your diet. You also want to limit trans fats, the kind found in foods made with hydrogenated oils, like margarine, crackers, cookies, and french fries.

> Boosting your HDL cholesterol level just one point can slash your heart attack risk by as much as 3 percent.

Limit your total fat intake to no more than 35 percent of your daily calories. Less than 7 percent should come from saturated fat. Keep your cholesterol intake below 200 milligrams a day.

On the other hand, you want to eat more soluble fiber, the kind found in oatmeal, barley, beans, apples, and other fruits and vegetables. Aim for 10 to 25 grams of soluble fiber every day. In general, you want to eat more fruits, vegetables, and whole grains, and less meat, cheese, eggs, whole milk, processed foods, and baked goods. Besides sticking to a healthy diet, you should also take the following steps to help lower your cholesterol.

▸ **Lose weight.** Being overweight increases your chances of having high LDL and low HDL levels — and a whole host of health problems. To get down to a healthy weight, you must burn more calories than you take in. That means eating less and being more active.

▸ **Exercise regularly.** Exercise not only helps you manage your weight, it also helps boost HDL levels. Aim for at least 30 minutes of moderate activity, such as brisk walking, every day.

▸ **Quit smoking.** This dangerous habit lowers HDL cholesterol and plays a major role in heart disease.

‣ **Reduce stress.** Researchers in London recently found that stress may raise cholesterol levels. Find ways to reduce or deal with stress in your life. Stress-coping strategies include exercising on a regular basis, listening to music, and practicing progressive muscle relaxation.

Even if you successfully stick with these healthy lifestyle changes, you may still eventually need cholesterol-lowering medication. But that doesn't mean you should give up on the healthy habits you've developed. They will help your medication work even better. You may also need lower doses of less-powerful drugs, which would lessen your risk of side effects.

Ask your doctor if statins are still right for you

"Old age is no place for sissies," joked actress Bette Davis. But when it comes to cholesterol-lowering medications like Lipitor and Crestor, old age may give you an unexpected advantage.

Are you a healthy adult over the age of 75? No type 2 diabetes or history of heart disease? Then you may want to talk with your doctor about stopping your statin.

When researchers studied healthy folks age 75 and up, they found that statins were not associated with a drop in heart attack and stroke rates. This has experts questioning the use of statins among older adults, who are more likely to experience serious side effects.

Your doctor might prescribe a statin if you have other risk factors like being overweight or having high blood pressure. So don't make any changes to your medications without talking to him.

Eat your way to healthy arteries

You know a healthy diet has a huge impact on lowering your cholesterol levels. But when you add these tasty treats to your menu, you might cut your cholesterol even more.

Artichoke. This centuries-old folk remedy contains a compound called cynarin, an ingredient now used in modern cholesterol-lowering medicines. But you can get it from the produce aisle in your grocery store. Just watch how you eat it. Dipping the artichoke leaves in a rich, buttery sauce will do your cholesterol more harm than good. Try a yogurt-based dip instead.

Fish and garlic. Fish, rich in omega-3 fatty acids, and garlic, full of sulfur compounds, team up to fight cholesterol. This dynamic food duo lowers your LDL better together than either one can do alone. A recent Indian study found that the combination of fish oil capsules and garlic supplements lowered LDL by 21 percent and boosted HDL by 5 percent. Serve up some garlicky fish for dinner. Your cholesterol — if not your breath — will improve.

Flaxseed bread. Why take Lipitor when this amazing bread works like cholesterol-lowering drugs but without the side effects? One study found that people who ate six slices of flaxseed bread every day significantly lowered their cholesterol. This remarkable bread is rich in soluble fiber and omega-3 fatty acids.

Walnuts. Full of omega-3 fatty acids, walnuts have been shown to lower cholesterol in several studies. Just don't go overboard. A handful a day should do the trick.

Regular cholesterol screening is important. Get a complete lipid profile, which includes LDL, HDL, and triglyceride levels, every five years. If you're at risk for heart disease or diabetes, do this even more often.

Grape juice. This artery-cleaning fruit juice is so powerful doctors are recommending it in lieu of drugs with none of their dangerous side effects. Both purple and red grape juice have been shown to lower cholesterol. That's probably because of quercetin, a flavonoid found in grape skins, which works like an antioxidant to prevent LDL cholesterol from building up on your artery walls.

Sidestep restaurant risks

You might have trouble sticking to your cholesterol-lowering diet when you eat out. But don't despair — here are some helpful tips for avoiding high-fat traps at restaurants.

- Italian. Stay away from Alfredo, carbonara, parmigiana, and anything stuffed or fried. Choose entrees described as primavera, piccata, marinara, grilled, or thin crust.

- Chinese. Avoid crispy, crunchy, sweet and sour, and fried dishes. Look for steamed dishes and ones containing these words — jum, kow, and shu.

- Mexican. Rarely eat nachos, chimichangas, guacamole, and taco salad shells. Fill up on fajitas, soft corn tortillas, salsa or picante, rice, and black beans.

Rise and dine with 3 heart-healthy power foods

Never had the opportunity to eat huevos rancheros? Qué lástima — what a shame! Rancher's eggs is a traditional Mexican breakfast of fried eggs over a warm tortilla served with zesty tomatoes, seasoned black beans, and creamy avocado — so yummy it has earned an enthusiastic following north of the border.

No big surprise there, considering the ingredients are tasty, filling, and packed with nutrients. Here's why these foods help keep your heart in fighting form.

Eggs deliver hard-boiled antioxidants. Historically, eggs took quite the beating when it came to heart health. But experts have changed their tune on the matter — egg-cellent news for your breakfast plate.

Why the change? It's not just that most of the cholesterol in your body doesn't come from the cholesterol you eat. Eggs are also a rich source of lutein and zeaxanthin, two antioxidants that may protect against heart disease.

Harvard Medical School researchers say one egg a day — the amount recommended by the American Heart Association — is safe for most people not at risk for cardiovascular disease. Just don't eat them with fatty foods like butter, bacon, and muffins.

Hot off the vine — tomatoes trim LDL. A small study of nearly 60 people with type 2 diabetes found that just two glasses of tomato juice a day boost LDL's resistance to the harmful effects of oxidation. Oxidized LDL, cholesterol damaged by chemical interactions with free radicals, is the kind most likely to lead to hardened arteries, heart attacks, and strokes. But lycopene — the pigment in tomatoes that give them their red color — may help prevent this dangerous cholesterol from forming.

In a separate but similar study, scientists gave 481 Japanese adults unlimited amounts of unsalted tomato juice to drink over a year. Most of the participants drank a little less than a cup a day. At the end of the study, the volunteers who had previously been at risk for heart disease saw large drops in their blood pressure and LDL numbers.

Avocado gets an "A" for plaque prevention. Penn State researchers have found that eating an avocado a day may protect your good cholesterol and fight the bad, artery-clogging kind.

The study recruited 45 overweight and obese adults who followed an average American diet for two weeks. Then, in no particular order, they each completed five weeks of a low-fat diet, a moderate-fat diet, and a moderate-fat diet with a daily avocado.

After five weeks on the avocado diet, participants had significantly lower levels of oxidized LDL than when they started the study and after completing the low- and moderate-fat diets. They also had higher levels of lutein, which may have prevented the LDL from being oxidized.

"Avocados are really high in healthy fats, carotenoids — which are important for eye health — and other nutrients," says Penny Kris-Etherton, distinguished professor of nutrition and author of the study. "They are such a nutrient-dense package, and I think we're just beginning to learn about how they can improve health."

Inside scoop on popular supplements

Many supplements promise they will lower your cholesterol, but not all of them live up to their claims. Here's a quick look at some cholesterol-lowering supplements and what you can expect from them.

CholestOff. This combination of plant sterols and stanols blocks cholesterol's absorption into the bloodstream, lowering LDL cholesterol but leaving HDL levels intact. Consider this supplement the 15-cent cholesterol cure — proven to work better than dangerous drugs. This pill has much fewer calories than other phytosterol-fortified products, like Benecol and other margarines. When taken as part of a healthy diet and active lifestyle, it could give your cholesterol an extra downward nudge.

B vitamins. Niacin and B12, two vitamins found in many dairy products, could help you avoid prescription drugs by lowering cholesterol, improving circulation, and even relieving depression. Niacin in supplement form can reduce LDL levels by as much as 20 percent and raise HDL by as much as 35 percent. Some strengths of niacin are available only with a prescription. Niacin should only be taken under your doctor's supervision.

Flaxseed. Lower your bad cholesterol levels with this natural supplement. It has no dangerous side effects and costs 50 percent less than leading prescriptions. Studies have shown flaxseed can lower cholesterol by as much as 15 percent. To take advantage of flaxseed's benefits, you must grind up the seeds — or buy them already ground.

CoQ10. This supplement does not actually affect your cholesterol, but it may come in handy to counteract the side effects of statins. According to researchers at Columbia University, people who experience muscle pain while taking statins have low levels of coenzyme Q10 in their blood. More research is needed, but perhaps taking supplemental CoQ10 can help protect you from muscle pain and muscle damage.

Guggul. This herb has received mixed reviews. While some studies show it lowers cholesterol, a recent University of Pennsylvania study found it might actually raise LDL cholesterol if taken in high doses. What's more, University of Kansas researchers found that guggul interacts with cholesterol-lowering drugs, including statins, making them less effective.

Attending religious services weekly can help extend your life almost as much as statins and exercise, according to a recent University of Pittsburgh study.

Policosanol. This supplement, derived from sugar cane, seems to be a sham. A recent German study found that policosanol works no better than placebo in lowering cholesterol. Previous supportive studies for policosanol were conducted by leading sugar cane producers in Cuba.

'No fasting' rule makes test — and your life — easier

Wouldn't it be nice if you could test your cholesterol without having to fast? That rumbly in your tumbly, as Pooh Bear would say, may be a thing of the past. New research out of Europe shows the test may be just as accurate when you don't go on a hunger strike beforehand.

The study, published in *European Heart Journal*, made an international recommendation that fasting is no longer necessary before cholesterol and triglyceride testing. Their research shows cholesterol and triglyceride levels don't change much whether you eat something ahead of time or not.

Talk to your doctor at your next visit to see if you can take advantage of this new rule.

Dollars&Sense
Get the inside scoop on the FDA

One of the main jobs of the Food and Drug Administration (FDA) is to regulate prescription and over-the-counter drugs. Drug companies can't even think of selling a new treatment until they test it extensively and prove to the FDA that it is safe and effective.

The road to FDA approval is long and expensive. Drug companies spend an average of 10 years testing compounds in the laboratory, then in animals, and finally in people before they can even ask for permission to sell a drug. Then, the FDA goes through a lengthy review process, looking at the evidence from studies to decide if a new drug's benefits outweigh its risks.

For every medicine the FDA approves, thousands more never make it. Only about five out of every 5,000 chemical compounds tested in the lab eventually get tested in people. Odds are, only one of those five will be safe and effective enough to get approved for sale.

The FDA's drug review process is considered the gold standard throughout the world. Still, it has problems, as recalls of high-profile drugs like Vioxx show. A drug can seem safe in studies but turn out to cause additional — and more serious — side effects once more people start taking it. Until a medicine goes on the market, experts don't always know just how safe it really is.

That's why you should stay actively involved in your health care. Question your doctor when he prescribes a new medication. Find out the facts and fine print about the latest "wonder" drug advertised on television.

IBD

Secrets for managing distressing symptoms

Your immune system could be making you sick. Although scientists aren't certain what causes inflammatory bowel disease (IBD), they suspect a faulty immune system could trigger inflammation in your intestinal walls. That causes frequent and sometimes bloody diarrhea, abdominal pain, and other symptoms that flare up and then fade — until the next flare-up.

The two main kinds of IBD are Crohn's disease (CD) and ulcerative colitis (UC). CD can affect your entire digestive system, whereas UC affects your large intestine, or colon.

Reaching a diagnosis can take many months and tests because IBD symptoms mimic other conditions, like appendicitis. Researchers say genetics play a role, so you're more likely to have it if someone else in your family has it. While there's no cure for IBD, there are many effective treatments and self-help strategies.

Explore natural remedies for less

Work with your doctor to find out which of these remedies could help relieve your symptoms. Then learn how to buy them for less.

Fish oil. Although steroid drugs are powerful anti-inflammatories, they can have serious side effects. Fish oil contains natural anti-inflammatories called omega-3 fatty acids. Scientists say fish oil supplements may help prevent CD relapses and reduce the amount of steroids needed to control UC symptoms.

Zinc. This important mineral fights inflammation and promotes healing. Ask your doctor whether you need zinc supplements, especially if you have Crohn's. Zinc deficiency may raise your risk of fistulas — abnormal passageways between organs caused by infection, inflammation, injury, or surgery.

Research suggests people with IBD are at higher risk for certain illnesses. Ask your doctor if you need screenings for osteoporosis, anemia, colon cancer, or other conditions connected with IBD.

Folic acid. Ask your doctor about folic acid supplements if you take methotrexate, an immune system suppressor that blocks the action of folic acid. IBD may also hamper your ability to absorb other nutrients, causing vitamin and mineral deficiencies.

Psyllium. Doctors recommend psyllium, the active ingredient in Metamucil and Fiberall, for mild or moderate diarrhea. One study even suggested psyllium might cut UC flare-up risk as effectively as the drug mesalamine.

Curcumin. This compound gives the spice turmeric its bright yellow color. According to research, it may help fight inflammation in your intestines. You'll find turmeric, the main ingredient in curry, in many Asian and Indian dishes. Supplements are available for people who can't eat spicy foods.

Sulforaphane. Some scientists think a bacterium called *Mycobacterium avium paratuberculosis* (MAP) can trigger Crohn's. MAP can infect cows, which pass the bacterium to you through their milk. Once in your digestive system, MAP might trigger CD.

Although more research is needed, two scientists from Johns Hopkins University School of Medicine think the sulforaphane in broccoli might help kill MAP. Brassica Protection Products, the company they founded, sells sulforaphane-rich products, like Brassica teas and coffees. For more information, call 410-732-1200 or visit *www.brassica.com*.

Bromelain. Fresh pineapple contains an enzyme called bromelain. Some doctors report that bromelain supplements helped heal the colon lining of people with mild UC. Experts suggest using supplements because you might not get enough bromelain from fresh pineapple.

Talk with your doctor before trying these remedies. Some aren't safe for people who have certain health conditions or take medication.

If your doctor approves, you're ready to start looking for the best prices. The following companies may offer below-retail discounts. Call their toll-free numbers to order a free catalog or simply shop online.

▸ The Vitamin Shoppe — 800-223-1216 or *www.vitaminshoppe.com*

▸ Swanson Health Products — 800-824-4491 or *www.swanson vitamins.com*

▸ VitaCost — 800-793-2601 or *www.vitacost.com*

Just remember to play it safe. Call your local Better Business Bureau to learn more about a company before you buy from them.

Tummy troubles? Put out the fire with 2 superfoods

You don't want to miss out on some surprising foods that can help you fight IBD. In fact, these two treats could be the inflammation fighters your diet is missing.

Munch on mangoes to soothe inflammation. In a small study, researchers from the Texas A&M University Department of Nutrition and Food Science asked people with IBD to add mangoes to their diet.

The participants started small and, for eight weeks, slowly increased the amount they ate, to avoid shocking their systems with too much of this fiber-rich fruit at once. By the end of the study, they were up to 200 to 400 grams each day — the equivalent of one to two whole mangoes.

Researchers reported that eating mangoes boosted the levels of friendly bacteria in people's microbiomes, and reduced blood levels of endotoxin, a chemical in your body that signals inflammation.

The reason? Experts credit a specific polyphenol, gallotannins, in mangoes. These natural compounds are easily broken down and absorbed by your intestines. And in turn, your body is better equipped to quench inflammation.

Brew up some powerful protection with green tea. Thousands of years ago, tea was thought to be one of the most potent known medicines. Today, modern researchers are once again exploring tea's healing properties. They found evidence to suggest the polyphenols in green tea can help lower your risk of cancer, Alzheimer's, and other chronic diseases. Researchers even think this delicious beverage can thwart IBD.

Animal studies show promising results. A recent paper published in the journal *Nutrients* suggests green tea compounds can fight inflammation and relieve symptoms in IBD sufferers.

Experts think the most powerful polyphenol in tea is epigallo-catechin gallate. This natural chemical breaks down as tea gets older, so aged teas — like black or oolong — have less of it.

Before you bring out the kettle, you should know that cold steeping tea may be even healthier. That's because brewing in boiling water will destroy some of tea's natural antioxidants.

Promising drug-free remedy promotes healing

People with IBD often have very few "friendly" bacteria in their gut. These bacteria help fight inflammation and harmful bacteria — but only if you have enough of them. Here's a way to get more.

Probiotic foods, like yogurt and yogurt drinks, contain live bacteria similar to the good ones living in your intestines. Experts recommend up to 10 billion probiotic bacteria daily. That's about the amount in a cup of plain yogurt, as long as the label promises live cultures.

If you can't tolerate yogurt, consider probiotic supplements. Research shows that the supplement VSL#3 may relieve Crohn's, ulcerative colitis, and even pouchitis, a surgical complication. Ask about VSL#3 at high-quality health food stores and pharmacies or visit *www.vsl3.com*.

> To help fight inflammation and prevent symptoms, find ways to reduce and manage your stress. Slow, deep breathing is a good place to start.

Other probiotic supplements may help, too. In fact, one study of people with UC showed that those who got 18 billion *Lactobacillus GG* bacteria daily were no more likely to have relapses than people taking the drug mesalamine.

For the best value, remember these three tips.

- When buying yogurt and yogurt drinks, like DanActive, read labels and pick products that display the expected number of bacteria alive at the time of use, not the time of manufacture.

- Store probiotic foods in your refrigerator to extend their shelf life.

- Shop at discount stores, like The Vitamin Shoppe, to pay less for probiotic supplements.

Clever tactic pinpoints problem foods

Foods might not cause IBD, but some foods can ignite your symptoms or make them worse. Fortunately, you can expose these troublemakers with a food and symptom diary. Here's how.

Keep a detailed record of your symptoms, when they happen, what you ate, and when you ate it. Use that information along with the "likely suspects" list on the following page to help track down problem foods. Try weeding them out of your diet to see if your symptoms improve.

▸ Milk and milk products. People with IBD are often lactose intolerant.

▸ High-fat, greasy, or fried foods. These foods can trigger diarrhea, cramping, and gas.

▸ Dried fruits, caffeinated drinks, and high-sugar foods, like watermelon and grapes. They can promote inflammation.

▸ Alcohol, red meat, and processed meats. These foods can set off CD or UC symptoms. What's more, diets high in red meat and alcohol may triple your risk of UC relapse.

▸ Prunes, fresh cherries, and peaches. These fruits can act as laxatives.

▸ Bread and potatoes. Up to 40 percent of people with CD can't absorb these and other carbohydrates. If carbs are a problem for you, talk with your doctor.

▸ Wheat, oats, rye, and barley. These grains contain gluten, which can cause abdominal pain, gas, and diarrhea in some people.

▸ Tomatoes, eggs, and peanuts. These foods are common allergens. Corn can also cause digestive problems.

▸ Red pepper and other fiery spices. Spicy hot foods often ignite symptoms.

Fiber is important for good health, but make sure you choose your fiber wisely. In his book, *The Maker's Diet*, Jordan S. Rubin, a naturopathic doctor, advises against eating the insoluble bran fiber in grains and cereals. Rubin recommends berries, celery, fruits, and vegetables with edible skins, and other low-carbohydrate foods high in fiber. Other experts warn that cruciferous vegetables, like broccoli and cauliflower, may cause trouble, especially when eaten raw.

IBD mistakes even smart people make

Be careful with that glass of ice water, especially when your symptoms flare. Drinking an icy cold beverage can sometimes cause cramps, warns the Crohn's and Colitis Foundation of America (CCFA). Who knew, right? Here are some other little-known mistakes that could be standing between you and feeling better.

Guzzling the wrong sports drinks makes things worse. Canadian research shows that people with active IBD consume more sports drinks and sweetened beverages than people who are in remission. But watch out when your symptoms are flaring. Excess sugar from drinks can trigger more diarrhea thanks to the extra water that is pulled into the intestines. So what should you do?

Vitamin D deficiency is one of the most common nutritional deficiencies in people with Crohn's, but talk with your doctor before taking supplements. People 55 or older are more likely to experience bad reactions or side effects, including nausea, abnormal thirst, headache, and irritability.

The CCFA recommends sports drinks during a flare to help you keep hydrated — but only if those sports drinks are low in sugar. They also recommend watered-down fruit juice.

Watch out for foods with emulsifiers. Have you eaten any polysorbate-80 lately? You may laugh but you probably have. Polysorbate-80 is an emulsifier added to foods to give them the right texture and longer shelf life.

According to animal research, emulsifiers like polysorbate-80 may alter the bacteria in your gut, skewing the balance in a way that encourages inflammation in your intestines.

Earlier research suggests these emulsifiers may play a role in inflammatory bowel disease. Some experts advise people with IBD to avoid processed, high-fat foods because those foods often contain emulsifiers.

3 easy ways to prevent flare-ups

You can make simple dietary changes to help prevent symptoms and flare-ups. Start with the ones your body will tolerate, and talk to your doctor about the rest.

Rejuvenate with fluids. Drink plenty of refreshing water to keep your body hydrated. To avoid dehydration from diarrhea, try broth, soup, and vegetable juice. They provide potassium and sodium — electrolytes your body needs.

Replenish your proteins. When diarrhea depletes your protein supply, eat protein-rich foods like poultry, lean meat, beans, and rice. Fatty fish is also a good choice. Their omega-3 fatty acids may help prevent CD relapses and reduce the need for some UC drugs. Although some fish contain high levels of contaminants, like mercury, the Food and Drug Administration says most people can safely eat up to two servings a week of fatty fish, like salmon, sardines, and lake trout.

Hamper IBD's henchmen. Some researchers believe unstable molecules called free radicals play a role in IBD and its severity. But antioxidants like selenium, vitamin C, and vitamin E may render free radicals harmless. Eat foods rich in these powerful nutrients.

And remember this. It's not just what you eat, but how. Switch from three large meals to six smaller ones spread throughout the day. You may be surprised at the difference it makes.

Incontinence

Can't-miss tips for a leaky bladder

Over 200 million people have loss of bladder control, or urinary incontinence (UI). Many of them find the situation so embarrassing, they won't even tell their doctors. Women are more often affected than men. In fact, six out of every seven adult cases of UI occur in women. The female anatomy, as well as pregnancy, childbirth, and menopause, contribute to the problem.

There are two main types of UI — stress incontinence and urge incontinence. When you have stress incontinence, urine escapes because of weak pelvic muscles and sudden pressure on your bladder. Laughing, exercising, sneezing, and coughing can trigger it. With urge incontinence, the need to urinate comes faster than you can get to a toilet. This type is more common in the elderly.

See your doctor if you have bladder control problems. He can suggest simple behavioral strategies as a first-line defense or prescribe medication to help you.

Super strategy for better bladder control

Simple exercises called Kegels are a great way to strengthen the pelvic floor muscles that control urine flow. More than 75 percent of women participating in a pelvic muscle training study reported improvement in their urinary incontinence symptoms.

The most important part of doing Kegels is locating the correct muscles to contract. Here's how to start. Sit comfortably with your legs uncrossed and your buttocks, abdominal, and thigh muscles relaxed. Remember to breathe normally. Next, pretend you are trying to stop urinating. Keep these muscles tense for about 10 seconds, then relax. Repeat this tensing and relaxing 10 times, three times a day. To really strengthen these muscles, try three different positions — lying, sitting, and standing.

When you're doing Kegels, don't tighten your leg, stomach, or other muscles. This can put pressure on the muscles that control your bladder. If you aren't sure you're exercising the right muscles, ask your doctor or other health professional for help.

Kegels help in other ways, too. To keep stress incontinence under control, tighten your pelvic floor muscles just before lifting or doing other things that cause urine leakage, like coughing and sneezing. When urge incontinence strikes, do Kegels to help you get to the bathroom in time.

Soothe and protect your skin

When your skin comes in contact with urine for any length of time, it can become irritated or infected. Always wear undergarments that keep dampness away. If you have an "accident," clean the affected areas as soon as possible. Wash with warm — not hot — water and a cleanser designed for incontinence that allows frequent cleaning without drying out or irritating your skin. After bathing, use a moisturizer and a water-repellent barrier cream that protects your skin from urine.

Be patient. You may not see any improvement for six to eight weeks. Kegels, like any muscle-building plan, require practice, and doing them faithfully will pay off for you. Then again, don't overdo it. Overworking those muscles can cause pain.

Set a schedule to curb the urge

You can improve most cases of urinary incontinence by using self-help remedies. Kegel exercises are a good example. Another is bladder training, a technique designed to lengthen the time between bathroom visits.

Start out by going to the bathroom every one to two hours, whether you feel the need or not. As you gain control, gradually increase the time between trips until you are only urinating every three to four hours.

If you get an urge to urinate sooner than your scheduled time, stay where you are and wait until the urge passes. Then slowly make your way to the bathroom, even if you don't think you need to. Relaxation techniques, like breathing slowly and deeply, can help you control the urge.

One survey found that 64 percent of people with incontinence don't do anything about it. And most adults wait an average of six years before discussing symptoms with their doctor.

Instead of a set schedule, some people can learn to put off urination after they first have the urge to go. Start by trying to hold your urine for five minutes. After you master five minutes, go for 10 and so on until you reach the goal of every three to four hours between bathroom stops.

As with Kegel exercises, bladder training is not an instant fix. It can take three to 12 weeks before you see any improvement.

5 ways to halt a leaky bladder

It might surprise you to find out that what you eat and drink, as well as your lifestyle, can have a considerable impact on incontinence. Why not make a few changes to help you control your leaky bladder.

Maintain a healthy weight. Carrying around excess weight weakens pelvic floor muscles. That's another good reason to stay at a healthy weight. If you're already overweight, taking off some pounds might solve your bladder control problem. In one study, overweight or moderately obese women decreased their incontinence accidents by 53 percent following a three-month weight loss program.

> Women who have had a hysterectomy are 60 percent more likely to have urinary incontinence after they reach age 60.

Watch what you eat. Many foods can affect your ability to hold urine. Citrus fruits and juices, tomatoes, spicy foods, chocolate, sugars and honey, artificial sweeteners, and milk and milk products are known offenders. Carbonated, alcoholic, and caffeinated beverages — including tea and coffee — can also cause problems. Try eliminating one item a day over a 10-day period and see if it improves your symptoms.

Keep yourself "regular." Constipation contributes to incontinence, too. Eating fiber-rich fruits, vegetables, and whole grains — and drinking plenty of water — will keep constipation at bay. Exercising regularly also helps.

Stop smoking. Tobacco smoke affects your bladder and urethra, the tube that carries urine from your bladder to the outside of your body. In addition, smoker's cough places stress on your bladder, which can cause leaking. It's never too late to quit. Ask your doctor for help.

Check your medicine cabinet. Another cause of incontinence could be hiding in your medicine cabinet. High blood pressure pills, cold remedies, and other medications could cause problems. Recent studies have also found that estrogen, once thought to prevent incontinence, can increase your risk of developing it. If you already have a leaky bladder, estrogen can make it worse.

Talk to your doctor or pharmacist if you think medication you are taking could be causing bladder control problems. Just remember — never stop taking a drug your doctor prescribed without his approval.

Why you need to drink more water

Don't try to control your incontinence by drinking less water. Fewer fluids concentrate your urine, which irritates your bladder and urethra and leads to more leakage rather than less. Stronger urine also smells worse and calls more attention to you if you have an accident. Some experts say you need two to three quarts of fluids a day. Be sure to stop drinking two to four hours before bedtime, especially if you are prone to nighttime accidents.

Limit saturated fat to keep your bladder in check

Steak, bacon, buttery biscuits — are these tempting foods a regular part of your diet? If so, you're like most people who eat way too much saturated fat compared to polyunsaturated fat. And that could be one of your problems.

In a study of 2,060 women, scientists found that women who ate over twice the amount of saturated fat as polyunsaturated fat were more likely to suffer urinary incontinence. And the more fatty foods they ate, the more severe their incontinence.

Researchers think that overloading your diet with saturated fat may contribute to bladder inflammation, one cause of urge incontinence. Foods like beef, pork, cheese, whole milk, butter, and palm oil are high in saturated fat, so try to limit those. At the same time, balance your meals and snacks with polyunsaturated-fat foods like fatty fish, flaxseed, walnuts, and sunflower seeds.

What to expect from your doctor

Urinary incontinence is not a consequence of aging, and nearly everyone with a bladder control problem can be helped. Unfortunately, less than half of the people with incontinence tell their doctors, and two-thirds of doctors don't ask their patients about it. Many doctors are as embarrassed as their patients to talk about it, or they don't know how to treat it. If this is the case, ask your doctor to refer you to a urologist or urogynecologist. Both types of doctor specialize in treating bladder and urinary problems, but a urogynecologist only treats women.

The doctor will ask you for your medical history. Make sure you tell him about any past and present health problems and surgeries. Also, be prepared to give him the following information:

▸ when the problem first started

▸ how frequently you urinate

▸ the amount of fluids you take in every day

▸ how often you drink alcoholic or caffeinated beverages

▸ what you are doing when you have urine leakage

▸ names of medications you are taking

You can also expect a physical examination and several tests to determine the health of your urinary tract. If your doctor diagnoses your condition as urinary incontinence, he will probably suggest one of these treatments.

Behavioral techniques. Pelvic floor muscle exercises, or Kegels, and bladder training are usually the first line of treatment.

Medication. Your doctor may also prescribe medication to relax an overactive bladder or tighten the sphincter muscles that keep your bladder closed.

Surgery. If conservative treatments fail, your doctor might suggest one of nearly 200 surgical procedures. To choose the best one for you, he will consider the cause of your incontinence, including any physical abnormalities in your bladder or urethra. Surgery to treat incontinence is usually safe and effective. Just be sure to pick your surgeon wisely. In general, the more times a surgeon has performed the procedure, the safer for you.

Alternative treatments. Ask your doctor if one of these treatments could help you.

▸ an injection of certain materials into the urethra, which adds bulk for more resistance to urine flow

▸ a medical device, such as a pessary, urethral insert, or urine seal, inserted to prevent leaks

▸ mild electrical pulses to stimulate the nerves that control bladder function

Secrets for staying dry

Don't let incontinence interfere with your lifestyle. There are many products on the market that will keep you dry — without anybody knowing.

Urge incontinence increases your risk of falling by 26 percent. That's because you're more likely to trip in your mad dash to the bathroom, especially at night.

You'll find absorbent pads and underwear at discount stores, drugstores, supermarkets, and medical supply stores. Shop around to get the best price. Become familiar with different products so you'll choose the best one for your needs.

Disposable inserts. These are worn inside your underwear and protect against small leaks. They resemble sanitary napkins or mini-pads, but they are much more absorbent and have a waterproof backing. Feminine hygiene products don't absorb urine very well. You can also get cloth liners that are held in place by waterproof underpants and can be washed and reused.

Adult diapers. Disposable protective undergarments for larger amounts of urine come in a variety of styles, sizes, and absorbency levels. You can get pull-on briefs that you step into just like regular underpants. Some are made from thinner, more absorbent materials and fit so it looks like you are wearing normal underwear. Be sure they fit snugly and have the right absorbency for your needs.

Reusable undergarments. Many styles of washable incontinence underwear look much the same as regular panties and briefs. They have waterproof panels and reusable liners. Newer styles have a unique design that wicks moisture away from the skin. They resemble normal underwear, but they are just as absorbent as adult disposable diapers.

Men's drip collectors. These are worn under briefs and are not noticeable with normal clothing. The pouch-like collector is made from absorbent material, has a waterproof backing, and fits over the penis. You can also buy washable briefs and boxer shorts with protective pouches that look and feel like normal underwear.

Insomnia

Drug-free sleep solutions

You lie in bed and stare at the ceiling. You toss and turn. You even try counting sheep. But nothing works. When you suffer from insomnia, bedtime becomes a nightmare. Whether you have trouble falling asleep or staying asleep, you're simply not getting enough sleep.

Insomnia does more than ruin your night and leave you tired the next day — it is hazardous to your health. Sleep deprivation not only raises your risk of having a car accident, it may lead to serious health problems, including diabetes, migraines, and high blood pressure.

Insomnia may be a symptom of another condition, such as anxiety or depression, or a side effect of medication. Make sure you and your doctor rule out these possibilities before treating your insomnia. Read on to discover the safest and most effective remedies to send you to dreamland.

Sleeping pills not worth money or risk

Prescription sleep medicine is big business, and seniors are most likely to take them. New products hit the market regularly, accompanied by expensive advertising campaigns and supportive studies funded by drug companies. But are prescription drugs for insomnia worth the money? A recent Canadian study suggests not. These popular meds cause memory loss, fatigue, even falls and accidents, and the benefits are "unimpressive." If they are in your medicine chest, you may want to reconsider.

Surprising effect of shorter sleep

Shorter sleep could mean a bigger waistline. Over a 16-year period, women who slept five hours or less per night gained an average of 2.3 pounds more than women who slept seven hours. They were also most likely to experience major weight gain — about 33 pounds. Those who slept six hours a night gained 1.5 pounds more than the seven-hour sleepers. Just one more reason to find a solution to your sleepless nights.

Natural ways to get a great night's sleep

Better sleep leads to longer life. But, despite what those ads for prescription sleep aids promise, better sleep does not have to come in a pill. Check out these simple, drug-free tips.

▸ **Stick to a sleep schedule.** Go to bed and wake up at the same time each day, even on weekends.

▸ **Stop lying around.** If you're not asleep within 20 minutes, get up and do something else, like read a book or browse through a magazine, until you feel sleepy again.

▸ **Keep your bedroom dark, quiet, and cool.** Consider sleep masks, earplugs, or heavy window shades.

▸ **Boot pets from your bed.** You love the furry little creatures, but they can disrupt your sleep.

▸ **Exercise by day.** Daytime exercise helps you sleep better at night. But don't work out too close to bedtime or you might have trouble dozing off.

▸ **Relax and unwind.** Don't bring your day to a screeching halt. Ease into nighttime. A hot bath may help.

▸ **Lighten up.** Avoid big, heavy meals before bed. You should also limit your beverages. Otherwise, you might have to get up in the night to use the bathroom.

▸ **Get rid of distractions,** like bright lights, a television, or a computer. Turn your alarm clock around so you won't keep staring at it.

▸ **Cater to your comfort.** Make sure you have a good mattress and pillow.

▸ **Put a cap on naps.** If you need a nap during the day, keep it under 30 minutes. Don't nap after 3 p.m.

▸ **Get some sunlight.** Spend at least 30 minutes a day in the sun. This helps control your biological clock and your body's production of the sleep hormone melatonin. If you have trouble falling asleep, an hour of morning sunlight may help.

If these lifestyle changes don't do the trick, try drug-free therapies. You can learn relaxation techniques, like slow, deep breathing. Or contact a sleep clinic and ask for information about sleep restriction and cognitive behavioral therapy — effective but costly treatments.

Turn on some music before you turn in. In a recent study, people between the ages of 60 and 83 improved their sleep when they listened to soothing music at bedtime.

Lull yourself to sleep with herbs

Sometimes the oldest remedies are the best remedies. The next time you have trouble falling asleep, try one of these five healing herbs that may work as well as drugs.

▸ **Valerian.** This is one of the most popular, effective, and versatile herbs for conquering insomnia. Drink it in a tea, swallow it in a capsule, or add five to 10 drops of the aromatic oil to a relaxing bath.

▸ **Chamomile.** Make a soothing cup of tea at bedtime to ease the stresses of the day. If you are allergic to pollen, however, choose a remedy other than this ragweed cousin.

▸ **Passionflower.** This flowering plant is particularly popular in England in preparations for calming the nerves. Brew a flavorful tea from the leaves and stems.

▸ **Hops.** Stuff some of these dried fruits into a small sachet bag or pillow and place it inside your pillowcase. Breathing the vapors from the alcohol in hops is probably what brings on the restful slumber.

▸ **Lavender.** To soak away your cares before bedtime, add a few drops of lavender oil to a warm foot bath. Or light a lavender-scented candle and enjoy the calming aroma.

Keep in mind that just because herbs are natural does not mean they are safe. The Food and Drug Administration (FDA) does not regulate herbs, so you can never be sure exactly what you are getting. Herbs may interact with medication. Always tell your doctor about any herbs you are taking.

Don't let jet lag spoil your trip

If a temporary change in your sleep schedule, such as traveling to a different time zone, leads to insomnia, your insomnia may only be temporary as well. Often, your sleep schedule will naturally return to normal. In the meantime, it may help to have your meals, go to bed, and get up according to the new time right away. And get outside during the day. Sunlight will help your biological clock adjust faster.

Rest easy with a simple supplement

You may not need potent drugs or mysterious herbs to get a good night's sleep. A dietary supplement may do the trick.

Melatonin, a hormone produced by the pineal gland, helps regulate your sleep-wake cycle. It kicks in at night, when it's dark, and promotes sleep. As you age, your body makes less of it, and a deficiency of melatonin may contribute to insomnia.

Fortunately, you can buy melatonin supplements — and millions of people do. However, experts disagree about the effectiveness of these pills.

One study found that melatonin supplements work best when your body is not producing melatonin on its own, such as in daylight hours. So it would help shift workers who sleep in the day or travelers with jet lag, but not most people trying to sleep at night.

Experts at the Massachusetts Institute of Technology say the amount of melatonin you take is key. And, in this case, less is more. They say small doses, such as 0.3 milligrams, work better than large doses, especially over time.

Keep in mind, the FDA does not regulate supplements, and the long-term effects of melatonin remain unknown. If you decide to try melatonin, take it up to 30 minutes before you plan to sleep.

Smart way to shush annoying snoring

Maybe you can't sleep because your spouse snores. Or maybe your own snoring startles you out of your slumber.

Here's an ingenious way to end the "buzz saw blues" without drugs or surgery. Simply sew a tennis ball into the back of your pajamas. This will prevent you from sleeping on your back, the position that makes you most likely to snore.

Northwestern University researchers found that regular physical and social activity helped older people sleep better. Go for a walk, then talk with friends while playing cards or board games.

Other surefire ways to stifle snoring include losing weight, avoiding alcohol before bedtime, quitting smoking, elevating the upper part of your bed, and sleeping on your side.

Snoring is often a symptom of sleep apnea. Talk to your doctor about this serious condition that is widely undiagnosed.

Snack your way to a good night's sleep

A huge meal right before bed may not be the best recipe for a peaceful slumber, but the right snack can help you get some shuteye.

▸ **Cherries.** Just a handful of tart red cherries, or some tart red cherry juice, might do the trick. Cherries contain a significant amount of the sleep hormone melatonin.

▸ **Cheese.** One study found that eating cheese at bedtime helps you sleep and leads to pleasant dreams. Of course, that study was conducted by the British Cheese Board.

▸ **Chili peppers.** A Tasmanian study found that those who regularly ate chilies slept better than those who didn't.

Another good bet is the combination of the amino acid tryptophan and carbohydrates. Tryptophan promotes sleep, while the carbohydrates help deliver the tryptophan from your bloodstream to your brain. Snacks such as tuna on whole wheat or cereal with milk give you a double dose of sleepiness.

Make sure to get plenty of calcium, magnesium, and B vitamins in your diet, as well. They aid in the production of melatonin.

On the other hand, you should avoid certain foods close to bedtime. Spicy, sugary, or fatty foods can interfere with sleep.

Are these foods zapping your ZZZs?

What's on your dinner plate may come back to bite you when you go to bed. That's because what you eat at night affects how you sleep.

A whopping 50 million to 70 million Americans struggle with chronic sleep problems. That's three times the number of people who live in Florida.

Women are twice as likely to suffer from insomnia as men. The risk of insomnia also increases with age.

When you toss and turn because you can't sleep, you're at higher risk for a slew of health problems like cancer, diabetes, depression, obesity, and high blood pressure. Not enough sleep makes you tired, grumpy, and even dangerous. Drowsy drivers cause 40,000 nonfatal injuries and 1,550 deaths a year, says the Department of Transportation.

Knowing what to eat and not to eat could mean the difference between a good night's sleep and a day full of fatigue. Here's what to avoid.

Skip spicy foods. Don't want to spend the night battling heartburn? Then hold the garlic, onions, and tomato sauce. Spicy fare can trigger heartburn, a fiery sleep robber.

And if you think you should reach for peppermint to put out that fire, think again. Some people use this refreshing herb to soothe an upset stomach, but it can also trigger heartburn.

Say no to that nightcap. Sure — that glass of wine may help you doze off, but forget about staying asleep. Alcohol is a powerful sleep aid, say experts, but it only helps you fall asleep for a few hours. After that, you will wrestle with your pillows for the rest of the night. It's because alcohol disrupts sleep homeostasis, your body's internal clock that regulates your sleep/wake cycle.

Cut out your nightly cuppa joe. It's hard to pass up a soothing cup of coffee or tea after dinner. But if you have trouble sleeping, you may want to switch to decaf. The caffeine in your brew can rev up your body for up to seven hours, causing a night of restlessness.

And it's not just the caffeine in coffee and tea. Remember to check labels for pain relievers and cold medicines for added caffeine.

Go easy on steak and fried chicken. You may be trying to fall asleep, but your tummy will be wide awake if you eat fatty or fried foods for dinner. Foods high in saturated fats take more time to digest, making your digestive tract work overtime, robbing you of hours you could be snoozing.

Bite into that BLT for lunch, not dinner. Bacon lovers beware — your favorite sandwich may be what's keeping you up at night. That's because those savory slices of pork contain tyramine, a substance that triggers your brain to stay awake and active.

And it's not just found in bacon. Eggplant, soy sauce, salami, tomatoes, and aged cheeses like Brie and sharp cheddar are also rich sources of tyramine.

Dollars&Sense
5 questions to ask about a new drug

Drug companies work hard to create new products to treat what ails you. But is newer always better? If you are thinking about trying a newly approved drug, first ask your doctor these questions.

Is it worth the extra cost? Television and magazine ads make the newest drugs seem almost too good to be true. But those ads — along with other costs of developing a new drug — mean a new brand-name drug costs more than older versions, and substantially more than their generic counterparts.

Is it better than old drugs? When a new drug receives Food and Drug Administration (FDA) approval, it's certified to be safe and more effective than a placebo. But the FDA does not compare new drugs to other treatments for the same condition. Discuss with your doctor the pros and cons of starting a new drug versus remaining on a well-established drug.

How long has it been around? New drugs have limited testing on certain populations, so sometimes side effects or dangers come to light after more people use the drug. The arthritis drug Vioxx, for example, was pulled after being on the market for five years. New studies showed that people who took the drug for 18 months or more doubled their risk of heart attack or stroke compared to those who took a placebo.

What does your doctor really think and why? Doctors, just like you, can be overly impressed with a new drug's promises. But sometimes a new drug may truly be better for your situation. Find out exactly why he is recommending it.

Is it covered by your health insurance? If the drug is not on your list of covered drugs, you'll need to pay for it yourself or file an appeal to ask your plan to pay for it.

Migraines

Reliable relief at your fingertips

Too many people with migraines don't realize they have them. The National Headache Foundation estimates more than half of migraine sufferers have been wrongly diagnosed with sinus and tension-type headaches. Maybe that's because most people think migraines always come with auras — flashing lights, dark spots, and other visual cues. But only one in five people see auras.

Diagnosing and treating migraines is critical. They can cause unnoticed mini-strokes, and women who have migraines with auras face twice the risk of heart disease, heart attack, and stroke as women without migraines.

Why suffer so much when new medicines and natural treatments can prevent attacks as well as ease symptoms? Stop settling for days filled with pain, and start living life on your own terms. You can do it safely without breaking the bank, and this chapter will show you how.

5 smart ways to fend off migraines

Certain things seem to trigger migraines, whether a poor night's sleep or a particular food. But you aren't at the mercy of these headaches. Establishing the right routines and eating habits can stop them from ever starting.

Set a sleep schedule. Changes in your sleep pattern, like sleeping in on weekends or going to bed later than usual, set the stage for migraines. Establish a regular sleep schedule and stick to it. Go to bed at the same time on weekends as on weekdays, and aim to get the same amount of sleep each night.

Eat right and regularly. Overweight and obese people are one-and-a-half times more likely to have chronic migraines. That could be due in part to poor eating habits. Evidence suggests a low-fat diet rich in complex carbohydrates, like whole-grain breads and cereals and legumes, cuts the frequency, duration, and severity of migraines. And don't skip meals — it lowers blood sugar, which can trigger an attack.

Track food triggers. Although no studies prove it yet, doctors and migraine sufferers swear certain foods set off headaches. Watch out for these common culprits.

▸ aged cheeses

▸ monosodium glutamate (MSG)

▸ processed meat, like hotdogs, made with nitrates and nitrites

▸ wine, dried fruits, and other foods containing sulfites

▸ beverages with tannins, such as coffee, tea, red wine, and apple juice

▸ beer and certain liquors

Keep a headache diary. Make an entry each time you have an attack, noting how long it lasts, the severity, and all food, beverages, and medication you took in the 24 hours before the attack, as well as what time you went to bed and woke up that day. Take your diary on doctor visits so he can look for a pattern behind the headaches.

Get moving. Exercise regularly to stay in shape and help relieve stress. Several studies show aerobic exercise, in particular, may help prevent migraines. Brisk walking and bike riding are good choices. Warm up first, since sudden, intense exercise can actually bring on a migraine.

Silence headaches with 8 sleep tricks

Daily migraines wreak havoc on your sleep, which causes more headaches. Making a few simple changes in your sleep habits can stop this vicious cycle, cutting down the number of migraines and their severity.

Sleep experts at the University of North Carolina asked 23 women suffering daily migraines to follow this advice each day.

- Do not take naps.
- Eat dinner at least four hours before going to bed.
- Limit the amount of fluids you drink for two hours before bedtime.
- Spend eight hours a night in bed.
- Go to bed at the same time every night.
- Do not watch television, read, or listen to music in bed.
- Use visualization exercises to help you relax and fall asleep faster. Thinking pleasant thoughts calms your mind.
- Avoid overusing headache medications.

After six weeks, these women had 29 percent fewer migraines, and their headaches were 40 percent less severe. After 12 weeks, more than half the women had only occasional migraines. The women who failed to follow three or more new sleep habits continued to suffer chronic migraines.

Thwart head throbbers with popular sleep aid

For some, the sleep hormone melatonin is a miracle cure for jet lag. Could it also heal headaches? Apparently, it can.

Just 3 milligrams battled not only tension headaches but migraines as well, show two separate studies.

▸ People who suffered chronic tension headaches an average of 20 days a month slashed those numbers down to, on average, just 13 days a month.

▸ Migraine sufferers also had fewer headaches when they took melatonin at bedtime. Over the course of the three-month study, their headaches were less intense, shorter, and didn't require pain medication as often.

Melatonin could help against headaches by working as an anti-inflammatory, regulating the brain chemical dopamine and the hormone serotonin, or by hunting down toxic free radicals.

Say goodbye to headaches with these stretches

Prevention is always the best cure. A team of experts in Italy may have found a way to halt daily tension headaches with a few stretches. They tested their techniques on more than 900 people. After six months of simple, daily stretches and posture exercises, people had fewer headaches and less neck and shoulder pain. Now you can practice these same tricks yourself.

▸ Sit in an armchair in a quiet room. Apply a heating pad to your shoulders and cheeks. Let your jaw drop naturally in a relaxed position. Do this for 10 to 15 minutes once or twice a day.

▸ Stand with your back, head, and hands against a wall. Pull your shoulders back until they touch the wall, then release them. Do this eight to 10 times in a row every two or three hours.

▸ Stand in the same position against the wall. Move your head forward, keeping the rest of your body still, then pull it back again until it touches the wall. Do this eight to 10 times every two to three hours.

- Place your hands behind your neck and lace your fingers together. Tip your head back while gently pulling forward on your neck until you feel a nice stretch. Hold this position for two or three seconds, then relax. Repeat this eight to 10 times, every two or three hours.

The more people stuck to the exercise schedule, the greater relief they felt. Help yourself remember to do the exercises by placing sticky notes around your house. For starters, stick one on your coffee pot, television, and bathroom mirror.

Fight back with a trio of powerhouse nutrients

Aspirin may be your go-to for pain, but you don't have to rely on it to banish headaches. Making sure you get these nutrients in your diet could be enough to ward them off.

Fight inflammation with vitamin D and calcium. Scientists believe anywhere from 45 to 100 percent of people who get migraines and headaches are low in vitamin D. In fact, that deficiency may help kick-start your headaches. It may also increase the frequency and severity of migraine attacks.

Chocolate may not trigger headaches, after all. Research suggests people often crave sweets before a migraine strikes. The craving, not the chocolate, may signal a coming headache.

Supplementing your diet with vitamin D may reduce both of these negative effects. Because it's an antioxidant and anti-inflammatory, this nutrient fights inflammation in your nervous system that could lead to — and worsen — head pain.

Low calcium levels may play a role as well. Vitamin D is

essential to calcium absorption, so lacking both nutrients may impact how often you suffer from migraines and how intense they are.

Make your life easy by eating foods high in both nutrients, like cheddar and Swiss cheese. If dairy triggers your headaches, canned salmon knocks vitamin D and calcium levels out of the park, too.

Migraines meet their match with magnesium. When a group of researchers analyzed multiple studies on taking magnesium, they found the supplements can significantly reduce the number of migraines you get. They've also reported that taking magnesium can make pain levels more tolerable.

The National Institutes of Health recommends 420 milligrams (mg) of magnesium per day for men and 320 mg for women. Since supplements above daily recommended amounts are common, use them under your doctor's supervision.

Looking for a way to add magnesium to your meals? Foods like rice and wheat bran, chives, and pumpkin and sunflower seeds are all packed with it and ready to knock out your headaches.

Herbal relief from your worst headaches

You woke up with your head throbbing. You know you should take your migraine medication, but you dread the side effects that make you feel even worse. What if you could lessen or even stop the pain without the nasty backlash? Here are two herbs that can improve your headaches the natural way.

Feverfew goes above and beyond to fight migraines. It's not often that a product can do even more than its name suggests. That's why feverfew is a superstar herb. Effective not only against fevers, it's traditionally been used to treat aches from head to stomach and has been especially successful against migraines.

▸ An aromatic and bushy plant, feverfew makes a helpful, although slightly bitter, tea. Its hydrating power is a great bonus since drinking too little water can give you a headache, too. If it makes your mouth feel dry or irritated, try using more water and fewer leaves or steeping it for a shorter time.

▸ Not big on hot drinks? Feverfew is available as a supplement, either alone or with other helpful nutrients. In a recent Italian study, scientists combined feverfew and other compounds into a "nutraceutical" supplement to combat headaches. The extra nutrients included magnesium, riboflavin, CoQ10, and an extract from a plant called green chiretta. After four months, this treatment significantly reduced the frequency and pain intensity of the participants' tension headaches and migraines.

Scientists think feverfew's anti-migraine activity is related to several factors, including its ability to block nitric-oxide synthesis and to release serotonin into your system.

How much do you need? Anywhere from 50 milligrams (mg) to a little over 100 mg per day is common in studies, but your doctor may recommend more. A typical over-the-counter supplement includes 380 mg of standardized feverfew. Check the label to be sure it contains at least 0.2 percent parthenolide, its active ingredient.

Get to the root of your migraine problem with ginger. Taking an herb that is as effective as a prescription drug may sound crazy, but it's true. When it comes to headaches, you could save hundreds with this homegrown solution.

Ginger's healing power can fix everything from motion sickness to vertigo. And against migraines, ginger works as well as the medication sumatriptan — without the side effects.

Both sumatriptan and ginger improved pain symptoms in a study published in *Phytotherapy Research*. The participants who took sumatriptan experienced side effects including dizziness and heartburn. But the only problem the ginger users faced was indigestion.

Just drop around 1/8 of a teaspoon of ginger into your glass of water at the first sign of a migraine to absorb the great results.

A hands-on approach rubs migraine pain

Migraine sufferers know all too well that these headaches can cause brain fog. It's impossible to concentrate on the simplest task when you're under attack from a migraine. Fortunately, regular massages may help keep those symptoms at bay.

And a specific type — known as a lymphatic drainage massage — may be the most effective. This treatment targets your lymph nodes, which help filter foreign cells and bacteria from your body.

Researchers recruited 64 women with frequent migraines and split them up into three groups. Some got a 30-minute traditional massage or lymphatic drainage massage once a week for eight weeks. The third group didn't get any treatment. The women also recorded how often they got migraines.

After the study was over, the researchers found that both massages helped cut down on the frequency of migraines compared to the control group. What's more, women who got lymphatic drainage massages needed fewer over-the-counter painkillers.

Talk to your doctor to see if this technique could be right for you. If you have congestive heart failure, an infection in your lymphatic system, or a high risk of blood clotting, lymphatic drainage massages could pose a risk to your health.

Smart alternatives bring sweet relief

Exciting new therapies are helping migraine sufferers cut back on expensive medications and live healthier, pain-free lives. Talk to your doctor to see if these options are right for you.

Acupuncture. Several strong studies have found acupuncture eases migraine pain and frequency. Experts think the needles may affect the way your brain processes pain. Other experts chalk it up to the placebo effect. Whatever the reason, it seems to work for some people. Discuss it with your doctor and look for a licensed acupuncturist.

Biofeedback. You can train your brain to stop headaches. Biofeedback and neurofeedback (EEG biofeedback) training teach you to control the physiological reactions, such as brainwave activity and muscle tension, that cause migraines, thereby short-circuiting the headaches early on. Look for a specialist certified in biofeedback or neurofeedback. Start by contacting The Biofeedback Certification International Alliance at 720-502-5829 or online at *www.bcia.org*.

Botox. Besides erasing wrinkles, Botox or *botulinum toxin* type A may treat migraines. In two recent studies, migraine sufferers who received Botox injections had fewer headaches and needed less medication to control them. People who had daily migraines and those who had had them for more than 30 years were least likely to benefit. Look for a headache specialist who has experience with Botox and expect to pay out of pocket, since insurance likely won't cover it.

Osteoarthritis

Great ways to manage your pain and budget

You're not alone if you have osteoarthritis (OA). Millions of Americans have this degenerative joint disease. In fact, it is the fourth leading cause of disability in the world.

Keep reading to learn about safe and effective treatments, as well as treatments with dangerous side effects, and how to get the most for your money.

Get wise to the hidden hazards of pain relievers

While many prescription drugs help relieve OA symptoms, some drugs have dangerous side effects. Vioxx, a member of the Cox-2 inhibitor drug family, was pulled off pharmacy shelves for raising heart attack risk.

Cox-2 inhibitors fall into the category of nonsteroidal anti-inflammatory drugs (NSAIDs). Many OA sufferers take NSAIDs for their arthritis pain. They're among the best all-around pain relievers in the world, and you don't need a prescription to get the over-the-counter variety — ibuprofen, aspirin, and naproxen.

But NSAIDs have serious drawbacks, too. At high doses, they can cause heartburn, ulcers, and gastrointestinal bleeding; increase your risk of heart failure and heart attack; and triple your risk of kidney failure. Older people with recent health issues are at the highest risk for dangerous kidney problems when they take this medicine.

When over-the-counter medications can't control OA pain, doctors may suggest a commonly prescribed opioid like oxycodone or hydrocodone. If you've ever taken one of these pain pills, you don't want to miss the astounding news that drug companies don't want you to know — they downplayed the highly addictive nature of these pain killers and even misled the public about their safety.

Opt for flat-heeled shoes next time you go shopping. They may not be glamorous, but studies show wearing high heels can eventually cause knee OA or make it worse.

Only take these medications at the lowest possible dose and under strict supervision by your doctor. Seniors also need to be extra careful with opioids because they can cause dizziness and drowsiness that could lead to falls.

Does this mean you should stop taking pain medications? Not necessarily. It means you should talk with your doctor about whether they are right for you — especially if you have a history of high blood pressure or heart disease.

Uncover common cause of joint pain

Could the medicine you're taking be the cause of your painful joints? Here are 15 drugs that cause joint pain.

- alogliptin (Nesina)
- atorvastatin calcium (Lipitor)
- dabigatran etexilate mesylate (Pradaxa)
- carvedilol (Coreg)
- conjugated estrogens (Premarin)
- febuxostat (Uloric)
- fluticasone (Advair Diskus)

- isotretinoin (Accutane)
- levofloxacin (Levaquin)
- linagliptin (Tradjenta)
- olmesartan medoxomil (Benicar)
- pregabalin (Lyrica)
- risedronate (Actonel with calcium)
- sitagliptin (Januvia)
- venlafaxine ER (Effexor)

Talk with your doctor if you think a prescription drug is causing your joint pain. Never stop taking a prescribed drug without his approval.

When you take heartburn medication with an NSAID, your risk of digestive problems goes down. Research shows that taking over-the-counter NSAIDs with a proton pump inhibitor, like Prilosec, carries a lower risk of stomach distress. Remember — always talk with your doctor before changing medications.

Maximize benefits from insurance plan

One in three Americans now uses unconventional therapies to treat their health problems, and 5 percent have used acupuncture to relieve pain.

Because alternative treatments are in such demand, more health insurance companies are willing to cover therapies like acupuncture, massage, and herbal supplements. The Centers for Disease Control report that a quarter of the adults who see an acupuncturist have either full or partial coverage through their insurance provider.

Take advantage of those benefits if you can. An eight-week study of people with knee OA found that acupuncture gave them twice as much pain relief as taking drugs alone, and there were no side effects. Although the benefits tapered off over time, if your insurance plan covers acupuncture, several months of relief might be worth it.

Glucosamine: The miracle joint preserver

Studies have shown that at least one arthritis supplement may work, particularly in relieving knee pain. Glucosamine is naturally found in your body and is a major building block of the cartilage that cushions your joints and keeps your bones from rubbing together. If you don't have enough in your body, your cartilage breaks down.

> Some arthritis sufferers have turned to an ancient practice called apitherapy — where a specialist injects bee venom into your body with an acupuncture needle.

By taking a supplement of glucosamine extracted from clamshells you may help repair that damage. Research shows these little pills may cut the pain of OA and preserve your joints. Some health professionals think glucosamine may even help restore damaged cartilage — something no other arthritis treatment can do.

While it may take a couple of months to see results, glucosamine won't bother your insides like NSAIDs. The usual dosage is 500 milligrams three times a day, but be sure to check with your doctor before starting this supplement. He can make sure it's an appropriate treatment that won't interfere with your other medications.

Best way to take pressure off your knees

The single most important thing you can do to relieve the symptoms of knee OA is lose weight. For every pound of weight you shed, four pounds of pressure is taken off your knees each time you take a step. If you lost 10 pounds, the load on your knees would be 48,000 pounds lighter for every mile you walked. That's heavier than three African elephants. No wonder your knees hurt.

Regular exercise will not only help you lose weight, it will keep your joints flexible and strengthen your muscles. Research shows that regular aerobic or weight training exercises will also lessen your pain and improve your walking ability. Balance periods of activity with rest — and vary your routine. Try fitness walking, water aerobics, weight lifting, swimming, cross-country skiing, cycling, or dancing. Just remember to warm up and start slowly.

And here's another great benefit — exercising three or more times a week builds up collagen producers in your knees, making them less painful.

If you aren't sure which exercises are right for you, ask your doctor to refer you to a physical therapist who can develop an exercise program just for you.

Helpful advice for people who use a cane

Hold your cane on the opposite side of your pain. Research shows it takes stress off your hips and knees better than walking with your cane on the same side as the painful joint. In fact, not using a cane at all is preferable to using it on the same side.

Ease arthritis pain with a delicious, vitamin-packed fruit

You don't have to pop pills to deal with arthritis. Try a tasty, natural remedy instead. Eating tart cherries can be a sweet way to soothe arthritis pain.

A Michigan State study found that, when it comes to treating arthritis pain and inflammation, tart red cherry juice was 10 times more effective than aspirin, ibuprofen, and naproxen — without the side effects typical of nonsteroidal anti-inflammatory drugs (NSAIDs). Anthocyanins, which give cherries their red color, contain anti-inflammatory compounds. That explains why cherries are so effective against inflammatory conditions like arthritis and gout.

In fact, cherries decreased C-reactive protein (CRP) and nitric oxide, two markers of inflammation, by 18 to 25 percent in one study.

> In one study, people with knee OA who received a ginger extract twice a day experienced less pain and required fewer painkillers than the people who received a placebo.

Long a folk remedy for gout, cherries actually help relieve this painful condition. At the first sign of a flare-up, eat about 20 cherries. You can also opt for dried cherries. Because their nutrients are more concentrated, you need fewer of them to get the same effect. One dried cherry equals about eight fresh ones. If you prefer your cherries in liquid form, here's how to reap the benefits of cherry juice. Mix 2 tablespoons of cherry concentrate with a cup of water. This should give you the power of about 50 to 60 cherries.

Cherries pack a lot of power into a small package. In fact, a 90-calorie cup of Bing cherries contains more antioxidants than a small piece of dark chocolate or 3 ounces of almonds. In addition to anthocyanins, cherries also provide the hormone melatonin, which also fights inflammation and oxidative damage.

You can always find ways to add more cherries to your diet. Just throw some dried cherries into your breakfast cereal, oatmeal, yogurt, salads, and pancakes. You can also add them to couscous, rice pilaf, risotto, and pasta.

Sip green tea for sweet relief

Not only will a warm cup of green tea soothe your soul, it will give your achy joints peace and comfort, too.

And that's because green tea is swimming in polyphenols — natural plant chemicals praised by doctors as useful for preventing and treating osteoarthritis.

Epigallocatechin gallate (EGCG), for example, is one polyphenol in green tea that controls inflammation. Others block the production of a compound in your body, nitric oxide. And that, essentially, stops your cartilage from breaking down. Polyphenols also protect your collagen, the connective tissue found in bones, tendons, and ligaments.

Not bad for a humble cup of tea.

Exciting new cure for knee pain

Your aching knees may get new life, not through surgery, but through the miracle of Botox, according to a study that showed the drug decreased severe knee pain 28 percent.

People who suffered from painful knee osteoarthritis experienced relief and improved function from Botox injections after just one month, researchers found. Those who received dummy injections showed no significant decrease in pain.

Although more research needs to be done, researchers are excited about Botox because it has the potential to replace knee surgery as an effective cure for osteoarthritis pain.

Cooling mint minimizes pain

Mint adds a refreshing zip to iced tea, fruit salad, and gum. But it may also provide a refreshing way to soothe arthritis pain.

Ancient Chinese healers used mint oil to treat injuries because of its anti-inflammatory powers and cooling effect on the skin, and ancient Greek doctors used cold-water compresses to ease swelling and joint pain.

Borrowing these tactics from ancient civilizations, University of Edinburgh researchers unveiled a new synthetic treatment with the same cooling properties of mint oil. Their study suggests natural "minty" compounds can work just as well as more conventional painkillers — without addiction or side effects.

That's because they're applied directly to the skin, lessening the risk of adverse effects. Unlike morphine, for example, which is not always effective for chronic pain, this minty treatment should work on arthritis and nerve pain.

Leeches may not be all bad. German researchers have found that leech saliva may have painkilling properties, and putting the little buggers on achy joints can relieve pain.

Here's why. The compounds act through a newly discovered pain receptor called TRPM8, found in some nerve cells of your skin. When activated by the cooling chemicals or cool temperatures, TRPM8 shuts off the pain messages to your brain. So it enhances your body's natural painkilling mechanisms. The new synthetic treatment combines the properties of mint oil with elements that specifically target TRPM8.

Researchers hope to further develop these special mint compounds into a safe, effective treatment for chronic pain, including osteoarthritis. That means more tests and studies.

But in the meantime, you can soothe your arthritis pain like ancient doctors with a homemade cooling, minty salve. Here's what you'll need:

- ▶ 1 cup olive oil
- ▶ 1-2 ounces beeswax
- ▶ 1-2 drops peppermint essential oil

Melt the olive oil and beeswax gently on low heat. Remove from heat and stir in the peppermint oil. Transfer the mixture to a clean container and let it cool completely. Store the container of salve in the refrigerator, where it should keep for up to a year.

Make sure to try it on a small patch of skin first to test for sensitivity. If all is well, rub it onto your skin, focusing on sore muscles and joints.

This topical mint treatment proves that pain relief doesn't have to come with a prescription. Now that's refreshing.

Make life easier with these clever products

You don't always need a pill to beat arthritis pain. You can find a variety of products made especially for OA sufferers. Whether it's a heat wrap to stop pain where it starts or a kitchen device that gives your hands a break, you're certain to find something that can make life easier for you.

Turn on the heat for fast relief. Go straight to the source of your pain and place a heat wrap on your achy joint. These devices can ease arthritis pain better than some over-the-counter drugs. Reusable wraps usually contain gel or beads that you warm in your microwave.

Some disposable wraps use capsaicin, the active component of hot peppers, or menthol to make the painful area feel warm without actually heating your skin. The sensation of warmth lasts about 30 to 60 minutes. ThermaCare disposable wraps use iron, oxygen, water, and salt inside cells that give off heat. These wraps come two in a box for about $6. The warmth from each wrap lasts about 16 hours.

> Capsaicin, the active ingredient in hot peppers, is an effective arthritis pain reliever. Capsaicin cream, made from dried cayenne peppers, is absorbed through your skin and works by deadening local nerves.

Disposables are more convenient, but they can get expensive if you use them every day — more than $2,000 a year. Luckily, you don't have to wear one all the time since the effects last long after you remove the wrap.

Make your home arthritis friendly. Pain isn't the only symptom of osteoarthritis. You have to deal with loss of joint function, too. It's easy to take care of that problem with a few helpful devices around your house. Have trouble opening jars? An automatic jar opener will have that lid off in no time. Can't reach shelves in your closet? Easily grab objects more than 2 feet away with a reach extender. Key turners, book holders, and doorknob levers all turn potentially painful tasks into pain-free ones.

2 tricks to adapt tools for arthritis

Arthritis is one of the most common conditions to develop as you age. In fact, over 50 million adults experience swelling, pain, reduced range of motion, and stiffness in their joints, prohibiting them from accomplishing a number of garden tasks.

If you are one of these people, don't let your arthritis keep you from doing what you love. These simple tricks will help you make the most of the tools you have and will help you keep gardening, despite your sore hands and aching knees.

Mozart and Bach can soothe your achy joints. A study found that listening to classical music eased chronic OA pain by distracting sufferers from their condition.

Grab the gloves. Though it isn't necessarily a way to adapt your tools, wearing a pair of padded garden gloves while you use your shovel, rake, or clippers may be just what your hands need. Gloves can relieve a lot of the stress on your hands, strengthen your grip, and allow you to use less pressure to accomplish the same goal.

Pad your handles. While the best option would be to buy new, lightweight, padded tools, you may not have room in your budget for a brand new set of garden tools, especially if the ones you already have can get the job done.

In that case, pick up some inexpensive foam pipe insulator wrap, and duct tape it around the handles of your tools. This will comfortably pad them and reduce the strain that comes from grasping the handles.

Dollars&Sense
4 ways to cut prescription drug use

Americans spend billions of dollars on prescription drugs each year. But do you really need all the drugs you take? You may be able to sidestep side effects and save money with these strategies.

Evaluate your situation. Don't assume you need commonly prescribed drugs. Here are some you may want to think twice about.

- **Antibiotics.** Just because you have an infection doesn't mean you need antibiotics. Studies show most ear infections and uncomplicated sinus infections clear up without antibiotics.

- **Statins.** These drugs, such as Lipitor and Zocor, work well to bring down high cholesterol, but their side effects may include muscle problems, liver damage, and memory loss. The lower the dose you can use, the better. Some research shows changing your diet may work nearly as well as drugs to lower cholesterol.

- **Aspirin.** Many people at risk for heart disease take a preventive daily aspirin. But people with a history of certain stomach problems are more likely to develop an ulcer from taking aspirin. This risk may outweigh the benefits for your heart.

Change your lifestyle. To help yourself live longer and avoid heart disease, try exercising and watching your diet instead of popping a pill. These simple moves toward a healthy lifestyle repeatedly prove most effective.

Check OTC options. Sometimes a prescription drug is a stronger version of a cheaper over-the-counter drug. For example, nonprescription Aleve is a less-expensive form of prescription Naprosyn. Ask your doctor to help figure out the correct dose.

Consider your changing situation. As you age, your drug needs change. Make sure you review your medications annually with your doctor. He should help you weigh each one's benefits and risks based on your age, health, and long-term expectations.

Osteoporosis

Fight for stronger bones

More than half of Americans over age 50 have osteoporosis, or they are in danger of getting it, reports the National Osteoporosis Foundation (NOF). What's more, you may have no symptoms until this sneaky disease causes a fracture in your wrist, hip, or spine.

Osteoporosis leaches away solid bone until it looks more like Swiss cheese or a lattice fence. This can lead to fractures, as well as loss of height, back pain, or a broken hip.

Although women get osteoporosis more often than men, men who break a hip have higher odds of dying within a year. Both women and men who fracture a hip are more likely to lose their independence. Start fighting back right now to prevent bone damage and its serious consequences.

Eat your way to tougher bones

Nab these nutritional tips to help keep your bones strong and healthy.

▸ Research has linked vitamin B12 deficiency to bone loss and fractures in older women. Get extra B12 from foods like fish, poultry, milk, and fortified breakfast cereals.

▸ High amounts of vitamin A from retinol, found in foods of animal origin, may boost your hip fracture risk. Get up to 40 percent of your vitamin A from beta carotene instead. Carrots, sweet potatoes, and apricots are good sources. Check your multivitamin bottle to see where your vitamin A comes from.

▸ The DASH diet for high blood pressure could help protect against osteoporosis, too. To get started on this mineral-rich diet, eat veggies, fruits, and whole grains daily. Limit salt to retain calcium. Avoid saturated fat but include calcium-rich nonfat or low-fat dairy products. Get some of your protein from oily fish, like salmon, which is high in vitamin D. For more information, visit *www.nhlbi.nih.gov.*

Hottest drinks for a healthy frame

What's better than a cup of coffee or tea to pep you up in the morning? The fact that a steamy sip of either can help secure your bone health.

Coffee beans are bone boosters. Orange juice may be the first thing that comes to mind when you think of acidic drinks, but coffee has acids in it, too. And lucky for you, they're good for your bones.

Caffeic acid, chlorogenic acid, and vanillic acid are just three of the acids found in your favorite cup of joe. Many of these acids behave like estrogen in your body. That means they can help improve bone mineral density and fight osteoporosis caused by an estrogen deficiency.

The sweet spot is drinking 2 to 3 cups. In a recent study of post-menopausal women, those who drank 2 or 3 cups of coffee a day

Caffeine could lower calcium absorption by a small amount. That's why the National Osteoporosis Foundation (NOF) says drinking more than 3 cups of coffee daily may hurt your bones. Luckily the NOF says you can help make up for any calcium loss from coffee and tea by getting enough of the mineral.

had a lower risk of fractures compared to women who drank less than 1 cup. But drinking 4 or more cups increased fracture risk.

Of course, drinking too much coffee has other drawbacks as well, like increased anxiety, headaches, and insomnia. So keep your intake in the moderate range to reap the most benefit.

Brew up a cup of tea to crack down on fractures. Feeling down in the dumps? A piping hot cup of tea is the perfect pick-me-up, but this old remedy can do more than help you feel better on a blustery day. Your tea leaves actually offer some serious protection for brittle bones.

In a recent meta-analysis, scientists pored over 13 studies that revealed just how powerful tea can be. The studies revealed people who drink tea tend to have stronger bones in their necks, lower backs, and hips than their non tea-drinking counterparts.

The secret lies with a naturally occurring plant chemical in tea called epigallocatechin gallate (EGCG). It works by increasing the activity of osteoblasts, which are the cells your body uses to repair broken-down bones. And it helps the osteoblasts already in your body live longer and work harder.

The studies don't recommend a single type of brew, but green teas tend have the highest levels of EGCG, followed by white, oolong, and black teas. If better bone health is your cup of tea, start sipping today.

Fend off fractures with vitamin K

Why take drugs when these delicious vegetables slash your risk of weak bones and hip fractures! Kale, turnip greens, broccoli, and spinach are all rich in vitamin K — a key ingredient for building and strengthening bones. Even better, research shows that just getting more of this vitamin helped cut women's risk of hip fracture.

But don't freeze K-rich veggies if you want their full value. Freezing destroys vitamin K.

And that's not all. Researchers have discovered a higher risk of hip fractures in men who take warfarin, a commonly used blood thinner, for more than a year. Scientists suspect warfarin affects the strength of your bones because it interferes with vitamin K.

Recent research suggests that supplements of another form of vitamin K might show more bone-fortifying promise than regular vitamin K. So keep an eye out for news about vitamin K2, and talk with your doctor to learn more. Meanwhile, you can get small amounts of K2 from chicken and cheddar cheese.

Breaking bad — weigh the risks of a drug holiday

Bisphosphonates? It sounds like a noise you might make when you sneeze. But they're actually drugs commonly prescribed for osteoporosis because they change the way your body breaks down and reshapes your bones.

Normally they keep your skeleton from breaking down too quickly, but there's a bit of a catch. These drugs also block your body from repairing teeny-tiny cracks in your bones. If you take them for too long, you're at risk for fractures.

The fix is really quite simple — after several years of use, stop taking the drugs for a while. Doctors weren't so sure how long you should be away from your prescriptions. But now new research says drug holidays shouldn't last more than two years.

Don't stop or start taking drugs willy-nilly, though. Talk to your doctor to develop a personalized treatment plan.

Snack your way to a stronger skeleton

Prunes — the fruit famous for improving digestion — rocketed into the spotlight recently when scientists discovered they may prevent bone loss in astronauts exposed to radiation. What, you've never been to outer space? That's OK. The next superfood of the fruit world can also help build bones in those of you who are gravity-bound.

> To get vitamin D from light canned tuna, buy the kind packed in oil. Canned light tuna in water is D-free.

No matter where you are — from Crater Lake to a crater on the moon — your skeleton is a 24/7 construction zone. A demolition crew breaks down old bone while a rebuilding team forms a new frame. As you age, the building group slows down. This is why older folks often have fragile, more breakable bones.

But prunes, or dried plums if you prefer, might be able to change all that. Researchers are surprised at just how much disease-fighting power they have. The bone-healing potential comes from three mighty nutrients.

Antioxidants. Prunes contain polyphenols that act as antioxidants to block bone loss and improve bone strength. Basically, they slow down the demolition crew and give help to the builders.

Vitamin K. At 28.5 micrograms per serving of five prunes, these sweet treats are loaded with K. The powerful vitamin teams up with nutrients like calcium to help build stronger bones.

Boron. No bones about it, boron is not as famous as its mineral cousin calcium. But it has an important place in bone health — extending how long vitamin D stays in your body. That's a big deal because vitamin D helps you absorb calcium.

Eat prunes, and you could build stronger bones in a matter of months, says a study partly funded by the California Dried Plum Board.

"Participants from our study maintained their bone mineral density by eating five to six dried plums per day," says Shirin Hooshmand, Ph.D., the lead researcher of the six-month study. "This can easily be achieved by snacking on dried plums or incorporating them into recipes."

Just eat a handful of these small, sweet fruits once a day. The best part — you may already have them in your fridge. Pair them up with other bone-building foods for a frame-fortifying diet. Try boron-rich fruits like raisins, peaches, and apples.

Defend bones with calcium

Get enough calcium regularly, and you'll be more likely to keep your bones strong and prevent a fracture. It's easy to get calcium from food. Start with low-fat dairy products. Add calcium-fortified versions of foods like orange juice, oatmeal, cereal, waffles, and energy bars. Top off by sneaking nonfat dry milk into recipes, and eat foods like kale, sardines, turnip greens, and salmon.

Just be sure you absorb the calcium in the foods you eat. A chemical called oxalate, found in spinach, rhubarb, nuts, chocolate, tea, wheat bran, and strawberries, can block calcium absorption. And dried beans contain phytate, a less-powerful calcium blocker. If you like these foods, just make sure you eat them an hour before or two hours after eating calcium-rich foods or taking calcium supplements.

Here's another smart idea. You can disarm phytates by soaking the beans for several hours, draining well, and cooking them in fresh water.

All that calcium won't do your bones any good if you aren't getting enough vitamin D. Your body needs vitamin D to absorb calcium. Salmon, fortified milk, and eggs are good sources.

Should you get screened for weak bones? The answer might surprise you

Do you know when to get your bone density tested? New guidelines from the U.S. Preventive Services Task Force (USPSTF) might shake up your thinking.

Bone density scans are quick, painless tests that can clue you in if you have weak bones or osteoporosis — before you break a bone. And if you've already been diagnosed with a fragile frame, they can let you know if your medicine is doing its job.

The USPSTF has long recommended that women over 65 get a bone density test. Now they say women under 65 should be screened, too, if they are at high risk for osteoporosis. Risk factors include smoking, drinking too much alcohol, being underweight, and having a family history of fractures.

Though the USPSTF only has official recommendations for women, men aren't off the hook. Experts say high-risk men over 70 should consider getting tested.

How to choose a better calcium supplement

Like most Americans, Mary tries to eat foods high in calcium every day, and — also like most Americans — she has yet to reach her recommended amount. If you're in the same boat, you may need to ask your doctor about taking a calcium supplement to fill in the gap. Use these guidelines and your doctor's advice to help choose the best calcium pill for you.

Pick a pill you can digest easily. Calcium supplements come in several forms, and each has its own advantages.

Calcium carbonate is the least expensive, but you must always take it with food to absorb it well.

Calcium citrate is easier for your body to absorb than calcium carbonate, so you can take it without food. Calcium citrate may also be right for you if:

> Worried you're not absorbing the calcium from your supplement? Drop one in a glass of white vinegar for 30 minutes. If it breaks down, the supplement will be absorbed well.

- ▸ you regularly take medicines for frequent heartburn or GERD. These may include histamine-2 (H2) blockers such as cimetidine (Tagamet) and famotidine (Pepcid) or proton pump inhibitors like esomeprazole (Nexium), lansoprazole (Prevacid), and omeprazole (Prilosec).

- ▸ other calcium supplements have caused constipation or bloating.

- ▸ you have a condition, such as inflammatory bowel disease, that keeps you from absorbing nutrients.

- ▸ you have low stomach acid, which is common in people over age 50.

Other forms of calcium, like calcium gluconate and calcium lactate, are expensive and aren't usually used to prevent fractures.

Look for a brand that's been tested. Find your ideal brand and product with these tips.

- ▸ Check for the U.S. Pharmacopeia or Consumer Lab seal to find a supplement that has passed independent quality testing.

▸ Beware of calcium supplements made from bone meal, oyster shell, or dolomite since some may contain dangerous lead.

▸ Check the supplemental facts label for "elemental calcium," the amount your body actually obtains from the supplement. Keep in mind your body absorbs more calcium if you take 500 milligrams or less at a time.

▸ Check whether your supplement comes with added vitamin D to help absorb more calcium.

▸ You may not need as much calcium from supplements if you already take antacids containing calcium carbonate.

If you're at high risk for heart disease, stroke, or kidney stones, or if you have a heart condition, stroke history, or kidney problems, ask your doctor if you can take calcium supplements safely.

Fun ways to fight bone loss

Exercise is a powerful weapon to strengthen your bones and reduce your risk of falls. Although you need 90 minutes of moderate exercise a week, you don't have to do it all at once.

Do some weight-bearing exercises — the ones you do standing up, such as gardening, brisk walking, or dancing. Weight training with light weights also helps keep your bones strong. If you'd like to chop your risk of falling and build balance, tai chi may help. Beware of high-impact aerobics, like step aerobics, because these exercises could increase your risk of fractures.

The less you snooze, the more you lose: Sweeter slumber shuts down brittle bones

BEEP. BEEP. BEEP. Few sounds are worse than a blaring alarm clock, especially if you spent all night tossing and turning. Restless nights set you up for a rough day, but they can do more than leave you feeling groggy. Skimping on shut-eye can actually cause your bones to start breaking down faster, leaving you at risk for a dangerous fall.

Get a great night's sleep to stave off bone loss. A recent study published in *Sleep Medicine* examined the sleep patterns of more than 1,000 men and women. Researchers found that those who generally slept poorly were also the most likely to have osteoporosis.

The reason lies with how sleep influences your sympathetic nervous system. That's the part of your nervous system that responds to stress by bumping up your heart rate and increasing blood flow. New theories suggest sleep disturbances may cause a jump in sympathetic nervous activity, which could egg on osteoporosis in two ways.

> You'll get more calcium from calcium-fortified orange juice if you shake the container before drinking.

- By boosting bone resorption. This is the process where osteoclasts break down old bone.
- By slowing bone formation. In this remodeling process, osteoblasts lay down new bone to reinforce your skeleton.

This bone-chilling combo leaves you at risk for fractures. And that's nothing to yawn at.

Clock more shut-eye to keep your skeleton strong. Shoddy sleep isn't the only thing that could hamper your bone growth. Not spending enough time in slumberland can also spur on osteoporosis. A study of more than 5,000 adults ages 50 and older found that getting less than six hours of sleep increases your risk of brittle bones.

Experts recommend seven to nine hours of quality sleep each night. Unfortunately, about 40 percent of American adults say they don't meet that standard snooze time.

Avoid falls and keep your independence

Falls are responsible for more than 95 percent of hip fractures that can lead to a nursing home or other long-term care, but simple changes around your house can help prevent falls.

▸ Put night lights near stairways and in bedrooms, bathrooms, and hallways.

▸ Use a rubber bathmat in showers or tubs. Add grab bars to walls near your tub, shower, and toilet.

▸ Give carpets and area rugs a skid-proof backing or tack them to the floor.

▸ Add ceiling lights to lamp-lit rooms. Keep rooms and stairs well lit.

▸ Keep kitchen cabinet items within easy reach.

▸ Clear loose cords, clutter, and low furniture from traveled areas that might make you trip.

Wise daily habits and smart medical decisions can help prevent falls, too.

▸ Wear low-heeled shoes with good support even at home. Consider thinner, hard-soled shoes. Athletic shoes may offer less stability.

▸ Avoid walking in flip-flops, socks, stockings, or slippers.

▸ Limit alcoholic drinks to no more than two a day.

▸ Sit on the side of your bed for several minutes before you stand. Standing up quickly can make you dizzy.

▸ Keep a flashlight by your bed.

▸ Have regular eye and hearing checkups.

▸ Use a cane or walker for added stability.

▸ Try hip pads. The new thinner hip protectors are worn under clothing, but they still help protect hipbones during falls.

Psoriasis

Don't break the bank handling this heartbreak

The red, scaly, itchy skin patches that show up in psoriasis affect around 7.5 million Americans. It's no wonder such famous people as singer Art Garfunkel; writer John Updike; and actor Jerry Mathers, "The Beaver," are among the sufferers. Statesman Benjamin Franklin, in fact, wrote of his trials with "the Scurff" over much of his trunk, arms, and legs, which a doctor's remedies failed to cure.

If you suffer from "the heartbreak of psoriasis," as the old television commercial called it, you may feel misunderstood and isolated. But you are not alone. The following potent remedies can help you spend less time battling the flakes and more time forgetting you have psoriasis.

Simple self-help offers hope for healing

In psoriasis, your immune cells mistake your skin cells for germs and attack them. Your skin churns out an excess of skin cells in response. This most often occurs on hands and feet but can happen anywhere on your body, including your scalp. It's more than just a skin disease, though. Up to 30 percent of people with psoriasis also develop psoriatic arthritis in their joints. Psoriasis raises your risk of diabetes, heart attack, liver disease, kidney disease, vascular problems, and chronic obstructive pulmonary disease (COPD), as well. The larger the affected area of skin, the higher your risk of these other illnesses.

Unfortunately, there's no cure. Psoriasis lasts a lifetime, flaring up during periods of illness or stress then dying down again. That doesn't mean you can't control the course of the disease. These simple tips will help you tackle the dry, itchy skin of psoriasis — and none of them involve spending money on expensive creams.

Scientists see a link between being overweight and suffering with psoriasis. Very low-calorie or vegetarian diets — even fasting — seem to reduce the body's inflammatory response so psoriasis flare-ups stay away.

Soak up some sun. Julie Moore, a dermatologist at Gottlieb Memorial Hospital, has some simple advice. "The sun is one of the best treatments for psoriasis," she says. "So in summer I encourage my patients to sit out on the deck and give their affected areas a good sun bath." It doesn't take much. Moore adds, "Twenty to 30 minutes is adequate to improve the skin; you do not need to sit out for hours."

Get cozy with gut bugs. Probiotics containing the bacterium *Bifidobacterium infantis* may help control psoriasis. These beneficial bugs may influence your body to make more regulatory T cells, special immune cells that rein in out-of-control immune reactions. Look for probiotic supplements that specifically contain this friendly bacteria.

Buy soft clothes. You don't want to chafe your skin with rough clothing.

Get your skin in shape. Exercise is one of the greatest natural healers, even for psoriasis. Skin, like all the other body organs, will be healthier if you exercise and eat a healthy diet. Good nutrition and exercise habits will keep your immune system functioning well, too.

Stamp out stress. The nerve endings in your skin release chemicals that control the immune cells living in your skin. Stress makes these nerve endings release more chemicals, and that, in turn, causes skin inflammation. Stress is one sure way to worsen your psoriasis. Gentle relaxation movements like yoga or tai chi may help.

Practice hands off. Don't scratch or pick at affected areas.

Keep your skin moist and supple. Buy a humidifier for your home. Your skin won't get so dry if the air is moist. Stay away from harsh soaps; cleaners; and long, hot baths. A warm bath with an oatmeal bath product will help heal your skin. Water- or oil-based moisturizers will soften your skin and help control flaking and bleeding.

Skip the salt shaker to save your skin

A bucket of popcorn at the theater may sound like a good idea at the time, but you may regret that salty snack after the movie is over.

That's because studies suggest salt may prompt several autoimmune diseases including psoriasis, multiple sclerosis, rheumatoid arthritis, and ankylosing spondylitis, or arthritis of the spine.

Yale School of Medicine researchers discovered the link between a high-salt diet and autoimmune conditions when they conducted an animal study. They say too much salt caused the animals to produce inflammatory cells closely associated with autoimmune diseases. These cells attack healthy tissue.

To keep your sodium intake down, try to cook from scratch so you can control how much salt is in your food. If you do buy prepackaged food, look for low-sodium options.

Improve your quality of life for free

The discomfort and pain of psoriasis, along with people's comments on your skin's appearance, can make psoriasis an emotional challenge. In fact, people with psoriasis are more likely than others to smoke and be overweight, maybe because they hide at home rather than lead active lives. Depression, embarrassment, and feelings of isolation can make it hard to meet new people.

Here's an idea you might want to try — join a support group for people with psoriasis. These small, informal groups often meet monthly and are open to people with psoriasis and their guests, like a spouse or caretaker. You can talk about the challenges of living with this condition, get ideas on treatments that work, and learn about the newest advances in drugs. Most importantly, you'll get to share with other people who understand what it's like to live with psoriasis. Finding a caring listener can help you cope with everyday life. You can find a support group near you through the National Psoriasis Foundation's Web site at *www.psoriasis.org*.

Attack psoriasis from the inside out

Psoriasis is more than skin deep. Like many skin conditions, it's related to your body's inner health and can be affected by what you eat. If you have severe psoriasis, seek your doctor's advice on the best treatment. But these supplements might help.

▸ **Fish oil.** Many supplements claim to fight psoriasis, but fish oil might really work. In several clinical trials, fish oil supplements improved symptoms of psoriasis, including scales, redness, and itching. Because fish oil is taken in large doses to get the desired effect, talk with your doctor before you try this treatment. As a bonus, fish oil, which is rich in omega-3 fatty acids, can help protect you from heart attack and stroke.

- **Turmeric.** This spice, the main ingredient in curry powder, is an ancient remedy for wounds and infections. Now, researchers are testing a chemical in turmeric — curcumin — to see how it can help other conditions, including cancer, arthritis, and psoriasis. According to clinical trials, turmeric can reduce the severity of psoriasis. It can be taken in capsule form as a dietary supplement or added to food.

- **Zinc.** People who have psoriasis lose more zinc through their skin than other people. Your body needs zinc to absorb linoleic acid, which is necessary for healthy skin. So, keeping up your zinc intake may be especially important if you have this condition.

- **Linoleic acid.** If you don't get enough of this fatty acid, your skin will become dry, rough, and blotchy. Eat plenty of foods rich in linoleic acid, like nuts, wheat germ, and vegetable oil.

Sweet relief from your pantry

For mild psoriasis, try making this economical, home-brewed mixture of honey, olive oil, and beeswax to treat scaly plaques. In a small study, this remedy helped clear up symptoms in 60 percent of the people who used it. Although in the study steroid cream was added to the mixture, when the amount of steroid cream was cut way back, it still worked.

Psoriasis balm

- 1/4 cup unprocessed honey
- 1/4 cup olive oil
- 1/4 cup beeswax

Melt beeswax in a double boiler over low heat, stirring frequently. Remove pan from heat and slowly stir in honey and olive oil. After it cools to a comfortable temperature, rub the warm mixture on affected areas of your skin. If you plan to store any leftover balm, mix in vitamin E from one gel capsule to help preserve it longer. Store in an airtight container.

Get wise to psoriasis myths

Psoriasis is one of the oldest known skin conditions. Although it has been around for generations, there's still confusion and mis-understanding about the disease.

> ▸ **Psoriasis is an old person's problem.** Most people develop this skin disorder before they reach 40 years old.

> ▸ **You'll always suffer from flaky plaques.** New treatments can do wonders to clear up the condition for extended periods of time in most people.

> ▸ **Scrubbing scales from flaky patches will make them disappear.** This irritation can make the plaques worse. Follow your doctor's advice.

> ▸ **Like father, like son.** Although psoriasis tends to run in families, having a parent with the condition is no guarantee you'll get it.

Magnesium salt: A mineral miracle for your dry skin

The Dead Sea — which is actually a lake nestled between Jordan, Israel, and the West Bank — is well-known for its healing waters. Rich in minerals, it has a long history of helping those with joint problems, breathing issues, and many chronic skin conditions, including psoriasis.

To test the truth in this tradition, researchers out of Germany had a group of people suffering from atopic dermatitis — a skin condition with similar symptoms to psoriasis — bathe in the Dead Sea waters every day for six weeks. At the end of the study their skin was significantly smoother, softer, and less inflamed. Experts give credit to the high amount of magnesium chloride in the waters.

Drinking coffee may reduce your symptoms if you take methotrexate or sulfasalazine for psoriasis. Researchers think coffee helps these drugs reduce inflammation.

Since a trip to the Dead Sea is out of the question for most folks, dermatologists sometimes use a similar, natural treatment of magnesium salt baths for their psoriasis patients.

If you'd like to give this a try at home, talk to your doctor, then look for bags or bottles of magnesium bath flakes. Just remember these two points:

▸ For the most benefit, make sure the product is at least 46 percent magnesium chloride by weight.

▸ And don't mistakenly purchase Epsom salt, which is magnesium sulfate, not magnesium chloride.

Dollars&Sense
Top 7 Rx questions to ask your doctor

When you visit your doctor, get the information you need to protect yourself from mistakes your well-meaning doctor or pharmacist could make — mistakes that could cost you your life. Ask him these seven questions about every prescription.

Bring a friend or relative with you if you are worried about understanding or remembering what he tells you. Write down your questions beforehand, and jot down the answers he gives.

▸ What are the generic and brand names of this medicine?

▸ What exactly is it for, and does it replace anything I already take?

▸ How many times a day do I take it? For how long? Do I need to take it with water or food, or at a specific time?

▸ Should I avoid any foods, drinks, or activities while taking it?

▸ What side effects might occur, and can I do anything to minimize them?

▸ Will I need to come in for tests or monitoring while on this medicine? How often?

▸ Will it interact with the other drugs, herbs, vitamins, and supplements I take? Does it contain the same ingredients as any over-the-counter pills? Are they safe to take together?

Once a year, bring all your medications to the doctor's office for a "medicine check-up" — including all prescriptions, over-the-counter drugs, supplements, vitamins, and herbal remedies you use regularly. Ask him to go over the dosage instructions, warnings, and possible interactions with you, and ask if there are any you can stop taking.

If you have trouble remembering your medication schedule, talk to your doctor about prescribing once-a-day versions of your medicines. You can even have him write out your schedule.

Raynaud's syndrome
Smart, inexpensive ways to short-circuit the pain

Raynaud's syndrome affects between 5 and 10 percent of the population — mostly women. It can strike out of the blue or stem from an underlying condition, like scleroderma, atherosclerosis, lupus, or rheumatoid arthritis. The attacks can be triggered by stress, holding a cold item, reaching into the fridge, or even air temperatures below 60 degrees Fahrenheit.

Raynaud's skews the way your blood vessels react to cold. Normally, cold makes blood vessels near your skin's surface narrow slightly to retain heat. In people with Raynaud's, blood vessels narrow dramatically. The resulting attack reduces blood flow to fingers, toes, and sometimes the nose, lips, or ear lobes.

As your skin turns white and then blue, you may feel pain, tingling, and numbness. In rare cases, lost blood flow may even cause tissues to die. Near the end of the attack, your skin turns red as blood rushes back in. Fortunately, driving back attacks may be easier than you think.

Stop an attack before it starts

Prevention is your best weapon in fighting Raynaud's. Follow these tips to lessen your chances of suffering painful fingers and toes.

▸ Spend more time indoors during cold weather.

- Wear layers of loose clothing to combat chilly temperatures. Include gloves or mittens, insulated boots, hat, scarf, earmuffs, thick socks, and a coat.

- Don gloves, mittens, or oven mitts before handling refrigerated or frozen foods at home or in the supermarket.

- Wear mittens and socks to bed on cold nights.

- Turn the thermostat up when using air conditioning or dress warmly, including a sweater or jacket, while in an air conditioned place.

- Drink hot liquids or eat hot foods before facing cool temperatures.

- Warm up your car before driving in cold weather.

- Talk with your doctor if you are taking beta blockers; headache drugs containing ergotamine, like Imitrex; estrogen; medicines with pseudoephedrine or other cold remedies, allergy medicines, or weight loss pills. These drugs can affect blood flow.

- Limit the use of vibrating tools and repetitive hand actions, like typing or piano playing.

If you are experiencing an attack, you can help ease the pain with these tricks and tips.

- Go indoors or move to a warmer spot.

- Soak your hands and feet in warm water or run warm water over them. Try rubbing your hands together or rubbing other affected areas to warm them. Thaw hands or feet with a heating pad.

- Swing your arms in circles or shake your arms and feet. Wiggle or massage fingers and toes.

- Don't smoke and avoid being around people who do. Cigarette smoke narrows your blood vessels, making your symptoms even worse.

Improve circulation with these nutrients

Recent studies suggest that if you have Raynaud's, you may need more vitamin C and selenium, a mineral found in unprocessed foods. Without these two important nutrients, you are more apt to suffer irreversible tissue damage.

In order to protect your fingers and toes, eat lots of citrus, cantaloupe, strawberries, peppers, papayas, mangoes, vegetables, grains, and organ meats like liver. A multivitamin containing an antioxidant formula would be a good idea, too.

Antibiotics help some sufferers

A recent study uncovered a connection between Raynaud's and *H. pylori*, the bacterium that can cause ulcers. After taking a week of antibiotics, 17 percent of those cured of *H. pylori* infection saw their Raynaud's symptoms disappear. Among those who still had Raynaud's, 72 percent experienced fewer and milder attacks.

Condition yourself for healthy blood flow

Fight Raynaud's naturally with a technique developed by Army scientists. People in a study held their hands in a bucket of warm water while standing in the cold for 10 minutes, three times a day. They did this every other day, for a total of 18 days.

At the end of the study, the people with Raynaud's had trained the blood vessels in their hands to stay open even when their bodies felt cold. The effects of this particular treatment lasted as long as two to three years.

Talk to your doctor before trying this remedy to make sure it is safe for you.

Savvy shopping secrets for cold weather

Stock up on cold weather clothes at after-Christmas sales or end-of-season closeouts in February or March. And don't forget to check sporting goods stores, ski supply stores, and even military surplus shops for bargains on battery-powered warming socks, winter clothing, and more. Consider battery-heated gloves, for example.

Meanwhile, remember these other shopping tips for clothing and accessories to keep you warm.

▸ Bypass cotton socks and choose wool, synthetic, or cotton-blend instead. These keep your feet drier and toastier.

▸ Look for chemical warming packets or pouches. Tuck the small ones into pockets, mittens, or footwear for long periods in the cold.

▸ Use a "coozie." Insulated foam bottle and can holders will help keep your drinks cold and your hands warm.

4 alternative treatments worth a look

Herbs and other nonstandard medical treatments may work for some people, but talk to your doctor first to avoid problems with side effects and drug interactions.

Fish oil. Two studies suggest that fish oil supplements show promise in helping improve circulation, but more research is needed before experts reach a definite conclusion.

Evening primrose oil. A small study found that evening primrose oil (EPO) supplements did not improve blood flow or temperature in study participant's fingers, but the supplements did reduce the number of attacks and weaken their severity.

Ginkgo. Two small studies suggest you might restore healthy blood flow to your painful hands and feet without drugs, vitamins, or exercise. The study participants, who took 120 milligrams (mg) of ginkgo every day for 10 weeks, showed improvements in blood flow and frequency of attacks. Just make sure you don't take ginkgo if you are taking blood-thinning medicines, such as aspirin or warfarin.

Biofeedback. Biofeedback uses devices to frequently measure body functions, like blood flow, to help you learn how to gain more control over that function. With practice, you may learn how to use your brain to help warm your fingers and toes. This seems to work for some people, but research has yet to prove its effectiveness. If you'd like to try biofeedback, ask your doctor where you can get training.

Pay less for supplements

If you decide to try supplements, mail order catalogs and Web sites may help you find a good deal. Call The Vitamin Shoppe toll-free at 800-223-1216 or visit them at *www.vitaminshoppe.com*. You can call Swanson Health Products at 800-824-4491, or shop online at *www.swansonvitamins.com*.

3 ways to stifle stress

Stress can make your blood vessels narrow just like cold temperatures can. Try these tips to calm your mind and your body.

▶ Contact your local hospital and other community organizations and ask if they offer classes in stress management.

▶ Talk to your doctor about starting an exercise program. If he approves, try walking, gardening, dancing, sports, or fitness classes. Exercising regularly fights stress and gets your blood flowing.

▶ Read and watch more funny stuff. Laughter fights stress and increases blood flow by widening your blood vessels.

▶ Pull out your old harmonica or any other instrument, and start playing. Lose yourself in the music, and let your stress slip away.

Cayenne pepper has a pain-relieving and warming effect on your skin. Sprinkle a little into your socks or gloves before you put them on. But first make sure you have no cuts on your skin. Wash your hands when you take off your gloves, and be careful not to touch your eyes or nose.

▶ You can cut through stress and boost your mood in just 20 minutes a week. How? Simply start a gratitude journal, and write about positive aspects of your life.

Restless legs syndrome
Wise ways to calm fidgety legs

Bedtime means darkness, quiet, and stillness — unless you have restless legs syndrome. Then you feel tingling, burning, creeping, crawling, or prickling sensations in your legs. Moving them relieves the symptoms, but it doesn't help you get any sleep.

Not surprisingly, restless legs syndrome often results in insomnia. This lack of sleep leads to impaired concentration and performance during the daytime. It can also lead to anxiety and depression.

Genetic factors, chemical imbalances in the brain, certain medical conditions, and some drugs may cause restless legs syndrome. This frustrating condition can also strike when you're sitting for long periods. It affects more women than men and is more common in older people. Although there is no cure for restless legs syndrome, there are things you can do to help you cope.

Simple tips soothe restless legs

When you have restless legs syndrome, you may feel helpless, but you're not. There are many ways to manage this frustrating condition — even without drugs. Try these tips to make your restless nights more peaceful.

▸ **Stick to a sleep schedule.** Go to bed and wake up at the same time every day. It's important to follow good sleep habits.

▸ **Sleep in.** If your schedule allows it, go to bed later in the evening and sleep later in the morning. Some people find that pushing back their sleep schedule reduces RLS symptoms.

▸ **Warm up or cool down.** A hot bath before bed may help. Cold compresses can also provide relief.

▸ **Get moving.** Mild to moderate exercise can help, but don't overdo it. Also, try stretching before bed.

▸ **Butt out.** Don't smoke cigarettes.

▸ **Make adjustments.** Find ways to accommodate your fidgety legs. For instance, sit on a high stool so you can dangle your legs. Or work standing up if you can.

▸ **Calm down.** Stress can contribute to restless legs. Try relaxation techniques or get a massage. Acupuncture has also been used to treat RLS.

▸ **Sock it to 'em.** Wear long socks to bed.

▸ **Keep busy.** Do activities like crossword puzzles or needlework when seated to keep your mind off your legs.

Pump up your iron to curb restless legs

Experts suspect a shortage of the brain chemical dopamine causes the symptoms of restless leg syndrome (RLS). But your body must have iron to produce dopamine. So if you don't get enough iron in your diet, you may not make enough dopamine either. In fact, up to 75 percent of people with RLS symptoms have low iron levels.

Not everyone who has RLS is iron-deficient. That means increasing iron intake may not help unless you are already short on iron, so talk to your doctor about testing your iron levels. If you have very severe iron deficiency, you may need iron supplements. But if your iron deficiency is milder, experts recommend you try to get more iron from food before you try a supplement.

To mine the most iron from food, use these tips:

▸ **Know the facts.** Iron comes in two versions — heme iron and nonheme iron. Your body can draw more iron from foods with heme iron. Clams and oysters are the richest sources, followed by organ meats, beef, pork, poultry, and fish. One easy way to sneak more iron into your diet is to add canned clams to your spaghetti sauce while it cooks.

▸ **Pair them up.** To absorb more iron from foods that only have nonheme iron, pair them with heme iron foods. For example, kidney beans only have nonheme iron, but you absorb more iron from them if they are cooked and eaten as part of beef chili. Other nonheme foods include pasta, dark green leafy vegetables like spinach and kale, dried peas and beans, seeds, nuts, and dried fruits.

▸ **Boost absorption.** Just 6 ounces of orange juice can double the amount of iron your body absorbs from nonheme iron foods. That means orange juice may help you calm your twitchy legs and get more sweet slumber. Drink orange juice with your cereal and milk, or eggs and toast. The vitamin C from the juice helps your body absorb nonheme iron from iron fortified-cereals, dairy products, breads, and eggs. Other good sources of vitamin C include cranberry juice cocktail, strawberries, sweet peppers, broccoli, oranges, kiwifruit, tomatoes, and tomato paste.

You can also up your iron intake by cooking your food in cast iron skillets. Boiling, steaming, or stir-frying food in any type of pot or pan may also enhance its iron content.

If dietary measures don't work, your doctor can prescribe iron supplements to get your iron levels up to normal. Take supplemental iron between meals and watch out for common side effects like constipation and diarrhea. Too much iron can lead to more serious gastrointestinal problems.

Give restless legs some rest

You may want to avoid sleep-inducing allergy drugs if you have restless legs syndrome (RLS). They can make your symptoms three to four times worse. Johns Hopkins researchers pinpointed the problem — diphenhydramine, the active ingredient in many allergy medications that calms histamine — the substance that makes you sneeze and itch — and brings about sleepiness.

It turns out that people with RLS have a higher number of histamine receptors in the area of the brain involved with the condition. When activated, these receptors affect nerve responses and also spark alertness or wakefulness. This promising discovery could lead to new treatments for RLS. But in the meantime, it's one more path to a restless night.

Eat right to sleep tight

Iron isn't the only nutrient that plays a role in restless legs syndrome. Deficiencies in other nutrients can contribute to the development of the condition, and some foods can trigger flareups. With the right choice of foods and supplements, you can take a bite out of RLS. Here's how.

Cut out caffeine and alcohol. They can make symptoms worse and hamper your ability to get a good night's sleep. Stay away from coffee, tea, cola, and chocolate — especially late in the day.

Elevate your E. Vitamin E supplements have been reported to help with restless legs syndrome. Aim for 800 to 1200 international units (IU) a day. You can also get vitamin E from vegetable oils, dark leafy greens, nuts, seeds, and wheat germ.

Make room for minerals. Calcium, potassium, and magnesium supplements may help. Food sources of these important minerals include dairy products, small bony fish, and legumes for calcium; fresh fruits, vegetables, fish, and legumes for potassium; and nuts, legumes, whole grains, dark leafy greens, and seafood for magnesium.

Fill up on folate. A deficiency in folate may contribute to RLS. Make sure you get enough of this B vitamin, which is found in dark leafy greens, legumes, seeds, and enriched breads and cereals. Folic acid supplements will also do the trick.

Run away from RLS

Many people who have RLS also have periodic limb movement disorder (PLMD), a condition that causes your legs to jerk involuntarily during the night. PLMD may lead to poor quality sleep, daytime drowsiness, and reduced alertness. Exercise can help decrease those nightly leg movements, a small Brazilian study found. The study compared two groups of sedentary adults with PLMD. One group did a single, intense workout, while another group completed 72 exercise sessions.

> Between 3 and 15 percent of all people experience restless legs syndrome. But among people over age 65, the estimated percentage jumps to between 10 and 35 percent.

Both groups had fewer leg movements during the night. However, the first group also became less likely to wake during the night, spent more of the night sleeping, and increased their REM sleep, the kind of sleep crucial to your learning processes.

Meanwhile, the second group fell asleep faster and spent more of the night sleeping than they did before they'd begun exercising.

Several conditions have been linked to restless legs syndrome. They may trigger RLS or share a common cause. These include osteoarthritis, varicose veins, obesity, diabetes, high blood pressure, rheumatoid arthritis, sleep apnea, and snoring.

Even if you don't have PLMD or RLS yet, exercise can help you lose weight and narrow your waist — and that may help prevent RLS. A new study found that people with a body mass index (BMI) score over 30 were nearly 1.5 times more likely to have RLS than those with a BMI under 23. What's more, people with the highest waist measurements were 1.5 times more likely to have RLS than people with the smallest waist measurements. More research is needed to confirm whether keeping a low BMI score and small waist size could help prevent RLS.

Rheumatoid arthritis
Ideas to improve your quality of life

Your immune system protects you from harmful bacteria and viruses. When you have an autoimmune disease, like rheumatoid arthritis (RA), something triggers your body to attack itself.

In RA, the membrane that lines your joints is the main target. The attack causes inflamed and painful joints, but it can wreak havoc on your whole body. Flu-like symptoms, like fatigue, low fever, and loss of appetite, are also part of the package.

Treating rheumatoid arthritis early can prevent damage. See a doctor as soon as you notice symptoms. It's possible you can take back your life from this debilitating disease.

5 great reasons to exercise every day

Exercise might not sound like a great idea when you have arthritis, but the truth is regular exercise will help, not hurt, your achy joints. Here's what exercising regularly can do for you:

- reduce pain
- improve joint function
- strengthen your bones

- build up your muscles
- help you feel good about yourself

Plan to get 20 to 30 minutes of aerobic exercise each day, as long as your doctor approves. If you can't manage it every day, just do what you can. A little is better than nothing. Avoid high-impact activities, like running and heavy weightlifting that stress your joints. Try these low-impact exercises instead.

Ride a bike. Cycling is a great way to work out without pounding your joints. A recumbent bike or a stationary exercise bike is your best option because it won't strain your knees as much. Stationary bikes are easier on RA sufferers with balance problems because they won't fall over.

If you already have a bicycle, you can turn it into a stationary bike with a cycling trainer, a piece of equipment you attach to the rear axle. The wheel will spin without going anywhere so you can cycle in front of your TV if you want. You can take it off when the weather is nice if you'd rather cycle outside.

You'll find indoor cycling trainers at sporting good stores or online.

Jump in the pool. Take a water aerobics class in a heated pool. Not only will the exercise strengthen your muscles, the water's warmth and buoyancy will help ease stiffness in your joints and reduce pain. In a new study, RA sufferers who took two water aerobic classes a week for 12 weeks improved their flexibility and endurance.

The Arthritis Foundation offers an Aquatic Program in pools throughout the United States. To find a program in your area, call the Arthritis Foundation at 800–568–4045.

When you exercise, recognize the difference between normal pain and arthritis pain. If your muscles hurt for a day or two after exercising, they are probably sore from working out. If your joints are swollen and feel warm when you touch them, your arthritis is flaring up. You might want to take a break or choose a lower-impact exercise. Talk with your doctor to come up with a fitness plan that works for you.

Eat your way to healthier joints

Your entire body is connected. This can be a good thing or a bad thing. Take rheumatoid arthritis. If your immune system goes haywire, your whole body feels the effects. The good thing is taking care of yourself and eating the right foods will help you feel better.

Mix in a little curry. Banish arthritis, not with powerful anti-inflammatory drugs, but with turmeric — the soothing spice you taste in curry. Ancient Ayurvedic medicine and traditional Chinese healers have used turmeric for thousands of years to treat inflammation. Now modern medicine has found evidence to support that practice.

> The upside to rheumatoid arthritis is you're 50 percent less likely to have seasonal allergies. But if you have both, the allergies may keep your RA from being as severe.

Turmeric prevented joint inflammation in animals with RA in a recent study, especially when they took it before the inflammation started. The secret ingredient is curcumin, a compound in turmeric that fights inflammation right down to your cells' molecules. Look for this spice at your grocery store and use it to perk up stir-fry or your favorite vegetables.

Make friends with flaxseed. Everyone agrees omega-3 fatty acids are good for you. And flaxseed has more than any other plant. This essential fatty acid can reduce inflammation, relieve joint pain, and reduce morning stiffness. Eating flaxseed to get omega-3 fatty acids is a cheap and easy way to take control of RA.

Take one to two tablespoons of ground flaxseed or one to two teaspoons of flaxseed oil to get these benefits. Ground flaxseed is easier to digest than whole seeds, and it goes well with other food. You can sprinkle it on cereal, mix it with yogurt, or bake it into muffins. Flaxseed oil works, too. Put it in cold foods, like salad dressings and smoothies.

Doctors aren't sure what causes RA. They think some people have an inherited trait that combines with an unknown factor, possibly something in the environment, triggering the disease.

Add color to your diet. When it comes to fruits and vegetables, brighter is better. Brighter colors mean more antioxidants, like carotenoids, that help fight inflammation and prevent rheumatoid arthritis.

Researchers found that oranges, bell peppers, pumpkins, tangerines, and papayas were full of the carotenoid beta cryptoxanthin, an antioxidant that lowers your risk of developing RA. People who ate the most of these fruits and vegetables were half as likely to suffer from rheumatoid arthritis. Just one glass of freshly squeezed orange juice a day will reduce your risk.

Arm yourself with antioxidants. What do vitamin C, vitamin E, beta carotene, and the mineral selenium all have in common? They may prevent rheumatoid arthritis. Studies have shown that not having enough of these powerful antioxidants in your blood can lead to RA. In one study, people with the lowest level of Vitamin C in their diets were three times more likely to develop rheumatoid arthritis. And the ones who skimp on vitamin E, beta carotene, and selenium are eight times more likely to develop RA.

Not sure where to look for selenium? You can find it in seafood, meat, and whole grains. Brazil nuts are also a great source. You can get all the selenium you need for the day by eating just two nuts — but don't eat them by the handful. Too much selenium can be toxic.

Sunshine vitamin shields against RA

Research shows vitamin D can help keep rheumatoid arthritis (RA) at bay. And if you already suffer from RA's achy joints, vitamin D might slow the disease's progression and ease your discomfort.

Boost your intake by spending 10 to 15 minutes in the sun a few times a week and drinking skim or low-fat milk. Or consider adding 500 international units (IU) of vitamin D3 to your daily regimen of RA medicines. In one study, people who did experienced greater pain relief after three months than those taking drugs alone.

Top pain-relieving remedy for stiff joints

Your body's immune system is always on the prowl for disease-causing viruses and bacteria. But sometimes your defenses get confused and attack healthy tissue. This is known as an autoimmune disease.

Rheumatoid arthritis (RA) is a condition where your body targets the lining of your joints. Rogue molecules break down the cushioning cartilage, resulting in throbbing, stiff, swollen hands, knees, or other areas. People with RA may feel tired, have occasional fevers, and generally not feel well.

Arthritis is the number one cause of disability in America. And you don't have to be a certain age. Three out of five arthritis sufferers are under age 65.

You've probably tried many remedies to ease your pain, from anti-inflammatory drugs to herbal creams. You may have even tried special diets. Recent research suggests that cutting out meat and focusing on plant foods may be one of the top ways to relieve your symptoms.

"A plant-based diet comprised of fruits, vegetables, grains, and legumes may be tremendously helpful for those with rheumatoid arthritis," says Hana Kahleova, co-author of a review on plant-based diets published in *Frontiers in Nutrition*.

Women are two to three times more likely to get RA than men. But they are less likely to report symptoms to their doctors, so they don't get the aggressive treatment they need.

"This study offers hope that with a simple menu change, joint pain, swelling, and other painful symptoms may improve or even disappear," she says. So what makes this diet so powerful?

▸ **It fights inflammation.** Meat and fat may increase your levels of C-reactive protein (CRP), a common chemical sign of inflammation. Studies say that switching over to meals loaded with veggies, fruits, and whole grains can cause those CRP levels to plummet. Plus plant-based diets are higher in fiber, which also helps keep inflammation at bay.

▸ **Fiber fuels the friendly bacteria in your gut.** A healthy microbiome ferments dietary fiber into short-chain fatty acids that fight inflammation. But the trillions of good microorganisms in your gut can only do their jobs if they're part of a healthy, diverse community. Want to keep your microbiome in tiptop shape? Eat lots of fruits, vegetables, and grains.

▸ **Going meatless helps you shed pounds.** Carrying around a spare tire increases your risk for RA symptoms. A review of studies found that people who lost more than 11 pounds were three times more likely to relieve their joint pain compared to people who lost less than that. And a plant-based diet is one of the best ways to lose weight.

So how can you get started? You don't need to cut out meat cold turkey. Begin with a few simple meatless meals each week, like veggie stir-fries or bean chili. And try to swap out beef and chicken for other protein-heavy foods, like lentils or tofu. If you start out slow, you'll find it easier to embrace a plant-based lifestyle.

Popular beverage cuts your risk in half

A cup of tea could protect you from the ravaging effects of rheumatoid arthritis. But don't count on coffee to do the same. Women who drank four or more cups of decaf coffee every day doubled their chances of developing RA, according to the results of the Iowa Women's Health Study. Researchers think a by-product related to the processing of decaf coffee could be to blame.

Tea is rich in antioxidants. It also helps to reduce swelling. The women who drank more than three cups of tea a day reduced their risk of developing RA by 60 percent.

Brew some green tea, too. Research from the Medical College of Georgia shows that green tea protects you from autoimmune diseases, like rheumatoid arthritis, because of the way it affects your immune system. Green tea lowers your levels of autoantigens, chemicals that trigger an immune response. Fewer autoantigens means your body is less likely to attack itself.

The leaves of green and black teas come from the same plant, *Camellia sinensis*. The difference is in how they're prepared. Green tea leaves are steamed right after they've been picked, which helps preserve the antioxidants. For black tea, the leaves are allowed to ferment. To make a great cup of tea, steep black tea and green tea for about three minutes in water that's hot but not boiling. Boiling water destroys some of the antioxidants.

Go for the heat to cool chronic pain

Move over pain pills. Capsaicin delivers topical relief that's hard to beat.

When you apply capsaicin cream to your skin, it zaps substance P, a chemical that tells your brain, "Ouch, this hurts!" The less substance P you have, the less pain you feel, especially if you suffer from arthritis, shingles, diabetic nerve pain, backaches, or psoriasis.

Sounds like a miracle cure, but capsaicin creams take some getting used to. Some people find the initial sting hurts more than their chronic pain.

As long as you don't suffer serious side effects like blistering or swelling, stick with it by rubbing a thin layer of cream daily with cotton balls or latex gloves. Steer clear of your eyes, nose, mouth, and private parts. Go ahead and wash your hands afterwards.

For achy fingers, massage hands with cream, but don't wash right away. Give the medication at least 30 minutes to work before rinsing.

Daily application will desensitize your nerves, but it may take up to two months.

You could opt for over-the-counter capsaicin patches sold at your local drug store or online. These have .025 percent of capsaicin, just enough to soothe sore spots for up to eight hours.

Or talk to your doctor about prescription patches. One study found just one patch with a high concentration of capsaicin, 8 percent, calmed nerve pain for up to 12 weeks.

Pamper yourself with touch therapy

Massage therapy is perfect for RA sufferers because it gets your blood circulating and eases pain, swelling, and muscle spasms. It also reduces stress, shakes depression, strengthens your immune system, and helps you sleep better.

Massage is no passing fad when it comes to healing. Your levels of endorphins and serotonin, compounds produced in your brain, shoot up during a massage to give you natural painkilling action. Your first massage doesn't have to be full of surprises. Here are a few things to expect.

▸ The massage therapist will ask you some questions to find out what kind of massage would be beneficial for you and to rule out any potential health risks.

▸ You will have a chance, in private, to take off your clothes and remove any jewelry. Only take off what you're comfortable with. She will give you a towel or sheet to cover yourself and keep you warm. The therapist will only uncover the areas being massaged.

▸ You'll lie on a padded massage table in a peaceful room. The therapist may play relaxing music. She might use lotion or massage oil during the massage to smooth out her movements. Tell her if you have any allergies to ingredients in oils or lotions.

▸ The massage will last between 30 and 90 minutes, but most sessions take an hour. The therapist will leave the room when she is done to let you get dressed.

An hour-long massage can cost anywhere from $65 to $80, but many insurance companies will cover some of the cost if you have arthritis. Look for a massage therapist at your local gym or YMCA.

Don't give arthritis a toothhold

A harmful bacteria called *Aggregatibacter actinomycetemcomitans (Aa)* has long been associated with the development of gum disease. And researchers now believe it can trigger an autoimmune response in people with rheumatoid arthritis (RA).

RA doesn't just cause painful and swollen joints. It can affect organs like your brain. In fact, many people with RA experience brain fog and have difficulty thinking. So what should you do? Keep your gums healthy by brushing gently twice a day, and get regular checkups and cleanings.

Dollars&Sense
Dodge dangerous drug interactions

Interactions between drugs, herbs, vitamins, foods, and over-the-counter (OTC) remedies can cause unpleasant side effects and even death. You can help your doctor and pharmacist catch dangerous interactions before they occur with a few simple steps.

Carry a list. Take a list to each doctor appointment naming all the prescription and over-the-counter (OTC) drugs, vitamins, and herbs you use, including creams and ointments. Note how much you take, how often, the condition each treats, and who prescribed it. You can get ready-made forms off the Internet. Go to *www.fda.gov/drugs/resources-you-drugs/my-medicine-record* to print out full-page medication forms. Another program, Vial of Life at *www.vialoflife.com* provides decals and medical forms to place on your refrigerator door to help emergency responders find out what drugs you take and learn your medical history.

Stick to one pharmacy. Try to fill all your prescriptions at one pharmacy, so the pharmacist can check for interactions. Each time you pick up a prescription, show the pharmacist your list of herbs, supplements, OTC remedies, and prescription drugs you take regularly. She may spot dangers the doctor missed.

Know food no-nos. Ask your doctor or pharmacist if you need to avoid any foods while taking your medication. Grapefruit, for instance, can interfere with 60 percent of oral drugs, boosting their strength to toxic levels. Avoid grapefruit and its juice while taking oral medicines and for 48 hours before starting a new drug, unless your doctor says it's safe.

Document side effects. Pay attention to how you feel after starting a new medicine. Write down any changes you notice, both emotional and physical, and share them with your doctor during the next visit. He may offer advice on how to lessen side effects or prescribe a different drug.

Avoid dangerous combinations

Food, herb, or OTC drug	Commonly overlooked interactions
alcohol	ibuprofen (Advil), naproxen (Aleve), acetaminophen (Tylenol), antihistamines (Benadryl), dextromethorphan (cough/cold remedies), tricyclic antidepressants, anti-diabetics, benzodiazepines (Valium), nitroglycerin, morphine, codeine, propranolol (Inderal), bronchodilators (albuterol), metronidazole (Flagyl), ketoconazole (Nizoral)
grapefruit juice, limes, pumellos, Seville oranges	anti-inflammatories (aspirin, ibuprofen), statins (especially lovastatin and simvastatin), calcium-channel blockers, estrogen, histamine (H1) antagonists, sedatives, erectile dysfunction drugs, amiodarone, immunosuppressives, cyclosporine, carbamazepine, saquinavir
St. John's wort	selective serotonin reuptake inhibitors (SSRIs), monoamine oxidase (MAO) inhibitors, digoxin, warfarin (Coumadin), sedatives, loperamide (Imodium A-D), imatinib, cyclosporine
ginkgo biloba	blood thinners, MAO inhibitors, digoxin, anti-diabetics
aspirin	alcohol, other nonsteroidal anti-inflammatory drugs (ibuprofen), insulin, garlic, ginger, ginkgo biloba
ibuprofen or indomethacin	blood thinners, steroids, aspirin, alcohol, some high blood pressure medicines
nasal decongestants	antidepressants
antihistamines	alcohol; cold medications; kava kava; sedatives; tranquilizers; sleep aids (Sominex); certain drugs for anxiety, depression, and high blood pressure

Rosacea

Attack common skin problem at first blush

Red in the face? Got more pimples than you did as a teenager? You may have rosacea, a skin condition affecting 16 million Americans that usually appears between ages 30 and 50.

Rosacea is most common among light-skinned women with ancestors from England, Scotland, Ireland, and Sweden — so common it's been called the "curse of the Celts." The red cheeks and bumpy skin of former President Bill Clinton, along with the enlarged nose of British statesman Winston Churchill, are due to rosacea.

If rosacea makes you feel more self-conscious than stately, your doctor can prescribe creams or pills to flush out the redness. You can also avoid common triggers, like heat, cold, and certain foods considered red flags for a rosacea flare-up.

6 ways to beat the heat when exercising

Strenuous exercise is good for your heart, but it's not so good for rosacea. A recent survey by the National Rosacea Society found that more than 83 percent of people with rosacea remembered having a symptom flare-up after a hard workout.

Everyone can get flushed from overheating during exercise, but it's worse for people with rosacea. To keep up your exercise routine without triggering a flare-up, try these simple tips.

Exercise in a cool place. During the summer, exercise outside in the early morning or evening when it's cooler. If you must exercise during the heat of the day, find an indoor gym or swimming pool to help you keep your cool.

Avoid the sun. Sun exposure can worsen rosacea symptoms, so walk, run, or bike in the shade. If you must be in the sun, wear a sunscreen with an SPF of 15 or higher. Avoid alcohol-based sunscreens, which can be irritating.

Go for shorter bursts. Rather than exercising for a full hour, divide your workouts into shorter sessions of 15 minutes. You'll get all of the benefits without overheating.

Lower the intensity. Instead of working at full capacity, go for less-strenuous forms of exercise. Your body will be conditioned, but your body temperature will stay in check.

> Household cleaners, especially aerosol or pump sprays, can make rosacea flare up, according to the National Rosacea Society. Use soap and water instead, or wear a mask when you're cleaning.

Keep your cool with a damp towel. Wet a small towel with cool water and wear it around your neck while you exercise. You can also find special towels that will keep you cool for several hours. Look for Frogg Toggs Chilly Pad Sports Towel or Cramer Stay Cool Sports Towel at your favorite sporting goods store or online.

Suck on ice chips or a cool drink. Cool your body from the inside out by keeping a bottle of cool water handy while you exercise. If you overdo it and feel flushed and overheated, cool down quickly by sucking on ice chips.

Smooth on minerals for natural beauty

Rosacea isn't a serious physical illness, but if you are a victim, it can take a heavy toll on your emotional health. In a recent survey, almost 90 percent of people with rosacea said the condition had damaged their self-confidence and self-esteem. It's not uncommon for people to miss work or shun social situations to avoid being seen.

To deal with unwanted redness, many people use cosmetics and other skin-care products. Unfortunately, these products often have ingredients that can make rosacea worse.

Not surprisingly, several manufacturers have designed makeup made of minerals for people with sensitive skin, including those with rosacea. These new cosmetics are composed of finely ground minerals, like zinc oxide, titanium dioxide, and iron oxide, with inorganic pigments added for color. Zinc oxide, the same calming agent in diaper-rash cream, may help with skin irritation.

Mineral makeup even offers a bit of sun protection, which is especially important if you have rosacea. The best thing about mineral makeup, however, is that it contains none of the usual makeup ingredients that can cause a rosacea flare-up — no fragrances, talc, preservatives, chemicals, or dyes. It won't clog pores or irritate your skin. That's why many dermatologists recommend mineral makeup for people with rosacea.

This remarkable makeup provides great coverage for redness. Some types go on a bit heavy, so take time to practice to get them to look natural. You can choose from foundation, blush, powder, eye shadow, and lipstick. Mineral makeup might cost a bit more than regular makeup, but a few economical brands are available.

Get the red out with light therapy

Erythema or red patches on the nose, cheeks, forehead, and chin cause the most distress to many people with rosacea. Antibiotics and creams work well on other symptoms, but sometimes this redness, which is caused by extra blood flow through the tiny capillaries, remains.

Dermatologists can treat this redness using several forms of light therapy — lasers, photodynamic therapy, and intense pulsed light (IPL). IPL, which has been available for over 10 years, is now commonly used. The treatments are done every three to four weeks, with the best results showing after four to six treatments. Combination therapy, joining light therapy with medicated skin creams and antibiotics, can help in severe cases.

Symptoms you should not ignore

Rosacea is not just a skin disease. It can also affect your eyes, causing redness, watering, burning, itchiness, dryness, sensitivity to light, blurred vision, and sties on your eyelids. You may be unable to wear contact lenses, and your vision may seem to get worse. More than half the people with skin rosacea also have these eye problems, called ocular rosacea.

You may think having bloodshot, watery eyes is only an annoyance, but ocular rosacea can damage your eyesight if you don't get treatment. Over time, it can lead to scarring of the cornea, the transparent tissue covering the front of your eye.

To treat ocular rosacea, your doctor might prescribe doxycycline or tetracycline, antibiotics used to treat skin problems. An ointment of erythromycin for the eyes and eyelids can also help take care of any infections. Cyclosporine ointment for eyes is a new way to treat the condition.

If you have ocular rosacea, ask your doctor if there's anything you can do at home. He might suggest using a watered-down solution of baby shampoo to wash your eyelids every day. If you have a stye — an infection of a gland on the eyelid — don't try to drain it. That will only spread the infection. Instead, hold a warm, wet compress, like a clean washcloth, to the stye for a few minutes several times a day until it heals.

Flush the stuff that causes flare-ups

Rosacea sounds like the name of a flower, and it may begin like the soft blush of a rose on your nose and cheeks. But when the bloom deepens and spreads over your face, the flower image fades quickly.

No one knows what causes rosacea, and there is no cure. It can be controlled, however. Here are some ways to limit the flare-ups.

Keep your cool. Anything that makes you flush — even saunas, the onset of menopause, or emotional stress — can trigger an attack of rosacea. In fact, a survey of people with rosacea by the National Rosacea Society found that for 91 percent of them, emotional stress led to flare-ups. The good news is 83 percent of those surveyed who tried stress management said it helped keep rosacea flare-ups in check.

Lotions and creams containing oatmeal may provide relief for rosacea sufferers by stopping itching and fighting inflammation.

Lower the heat. The "hot" in spices and the temperature of hot drinks and solid foods are among the biggest triggers of the symptoms of rosacea. To prevent heat from rushing to

What you should know about rosacea

Symptoms of rosacea	Self-help remedies
flushing, redness, visible blood vessels, scaliness, facial swelling (erythematotelangiectatic rosacea)	avoid excessive heat, cold, strenuous exercise, and trigger foods use mineral makeup or concealer
redness and pimples that look like acne (papulopustular rosacea)	wash face with warm water and gentle soap use a light, oil-free moisturizer
thickened skin, bumps, enlarged nose (phymatous rosacea)	treat rosacea at an early stage to avoid facial disfigurement
watery or bloodshot eyes, sometimes with burning or itching, sties on eyelids (ocular rosacea)	warm, wet compress several times a day, wash eyelids with baby shampoo solution seek treatment to avoid vision loss

your face, avoid foods with black and white pepper, paprika, red pepper, and cayenne.

It's the heat, not the caffeine or any other substance, in hot coffee or tea that causes problems. You should be able to continue to enjoy these if you reduce the temperature. Letting hot foods cool to room temperature before eating can help prevent a flare-up as well.

Watch out for these high-histamine foods. Tomatoes, eggplant, spinach, cheese, chocolate, chicken livers, citrus fruits, bananas, raisins, red plums, figs, avocados, yogurt, and sour cream are foods that are high in histamines or release histamines into the body. They cause flushing because that's part of the job histamines normally do. When a burn on your skin turns red, for example, histamine is the reason.

When your face turns red from flushing, it increases the skin irritations of rosacea. Try taking an antihistamine about two hours before a meal that includes these high-histamine foods.

Hold the pickled, smoked, marinated, and fermented foods. Problem-causing ingredients like vinegar, soy sauce, and vanilla in foods prepared in these ways are likely to cause symptoms of rosacea to return. Alcoholic beverages can also stir up an outbreak.

Say no to niacin and ban the beans. Flare-ups are sometimes caused by foods containing niacin, like liver and yeast. Breads made with yeast, however, seem to be okay for most folks. The pods of broad-leaf beans such as limas, navy beans, and peas sometimes stir up the flushes that bring on the roughness and redness of rosacea. Try taking an aspirin before eating foods that contain niacin.

Not everybody is affected by the same foods and beverages. It's a good idea to keep a diary of what you eat and drink to help you decide which ones affect your condition. You'll learn which ones to avoid, and maybe you'll find that you can safely continue some of your favorites.

Shingles

Get tough on a mysterious virus

A shingles outbreak, whether brief and mild or severe and lingering, always causes pain. The herpes virus known as varicella-zoster virus, which triggers chickenpox in children, is also responsible for shingles. If you had chickenpox, the virus hides in nerve cells and can reappear years later. Half of the population living to 85 years old will experience shingles during their lifetime.

Like chickenpox, shingles causes an itchy rash, as well as pain. True to its name, which means "belt" or "girdle" in Latin, a shingles rash forms a band on one side of the body and the blisters that develop take about seven to 10 days to scab over.

Pain can continue for weeks or months after the rash has healed. When the pain lasts longer than three months, it's called postherpetic neuralgia.

Cut your odds with fruits and veggies

Add pineapple slices to a ham sandwich, cranberry sauce to a turkey sandwich, or sautéed peppers, onions, and carrots to your spaghetti sauce. These changes not only add more flavor to your food but may also help you avoid shingles.

A British study found that people who ate one piece of fruit or less daily had three times as much risk of shingles as people who ate more than three servings of fruit every day. And for people over age 60, the fewer vegetables they ate, the higher their risk of suffering this painful condition.

Shingles risk also rises for those over 60 who take in lower amounts of vitamin A, vitamin B6, vitamin C, vitamin E, folic acid, iron, and zinc. The researchers suggest that age weakens your immune system and its resistance to the shingles virus.

> Shingles cases are increasing, possibly because most children in the United States are getting the chickenpox vaccine. That means less protective exposure to the virus for adults.

The British researchers suspect fruits, vegetables, and the vitamins and minerals they studied help defend your immune system against age-related weakening, making you less vulnerable to shingles. But this only works if you eat enough fruits and vegetables. Start by making small changes like these.

▸ Add shredded peppers and carrots to chili.

▸ Slip thin apple slices into a peanut butter or ham sandwich.

▸ Add chopped vegetables to canned chicken noodle soup.

Take action to outsmart shingles

It's not too late to fight back, even after you come down with shingles. Anti-viral drugs, which work by keeping the virus from reproducing, can help. They do the most good if you start taking them within 72 hours of your first symptoms. These drugs can make the shingles attack milder, help you heal faster, and possibly ward off the discomfort of postherpetic neuralgia.

Because younger people who develop shingles usually get well quickly with few complications, these anti-viral drugs are not usually recommended for them. Instead, they are most important for people with shingles who:

▸ are elderly.　　　　　　　▸ have a shingles rash near their eyes.

▸ have very severe pain.   ▸ have a weakened immune system.

▸ develop a shingles rash over a large area of skin.

See your doctor as soon as you have symptoms so you can take advantage of anti-viral drugs.

Help yourself to pain relief

You'll need to see your doctor if you think you have shingles. Once the diagnosis is confirmed, follow your doctor's orders and take some extra steps to ease the pain. To treat an acute attack of shingles — and all the pain and itching that come with it — try these self-help ideas.

Soak away the pain. Soothing baths help reduce itching for children with chickenpox, and they can help shingles sufferers, too. Pour one or two cups of colloidal (finely ground) oatmeal into a tub of warm water and soak for about 20 minutes. You can also try one-half to one cup of baking soda or a cup of cornstarch.

Grab an old standby. You probably have aspirin or ibuprofen in your medicine cabinet. These or other NSAIDs (nonsteroidal anti-inflammatory drugs) can help with the discomfort of a severe shingles outbreak.

If you have shingles, you can't give it to someone else. However, exposure to the fluid from shingles blisters can cause chickenpox in people who have never had it.

Quiet the virus with peaceful exercises

Want to silence shingles? Practice the steps of Tai Chi Chih, or "meditation with movement." This traditional Chinese style of exercise, adapted from a form of martial arts, was developed to help keep older people fit. It uses a series of slow movements and balance poses.

In a recent study, researchers in California found that seniors who participated in Tai Chi Chih classes three times a week for 45 minutes boosted their immunity to the virus that causes shingles. In the study, participants followed an instructor through a series of 20 Tai Chi Chih movements.

Surprisingly, shingles raises your risk of stroke by 35 percent and your risk of heart attack by 59 percent. The first year after having shingles is the most dangerous — your risk decreases with time.

After 15 weeks of classes, the exercisers were given a blood test. It showed certain immunity factors, which protect against shingles, had increased by 50 percent. People in a control group, who did not take the classes, had no change in these immunity factors. Along with keeping shingles at bay, the Tai Chi Chih classes also helped the exercisers with their everyday movements, such as climbing stairs and walking.

Zap long-term nerve pain

When a young person develops shingles, there are rarely complications. But if you're a senior, the virus can keep you down a long time. The rash will eventually fade, but the pain may linger for months or years. The virus drills tiny holes in your nerves to infect them, damaging them in the process. These nerves carry electrical signals that leak out through the holes, making the nerves misfire painfully. It's called postherpetic neuralgia (PHN). Fewer than one in five people with shingles develop PHN, but the older you are when you get shingles, the higher your risk and the more severe the pain will be.

PHN pain can range from tenderness to a constant burning or throbbing in a nerve. Some people become so sensitive to any sensation that even a breeze can cause pain.

If you suffer from PHN, you are not alone. Don't suffer in silence. Ask your doctor about the following treatments.

Lidocaine patch. The lidocaine patch is one of the newest treatments for PHN. Lidocaine is an ingredient often found in products that relieve sunburn and other skin pain. Now researchers have developed large, lidocaine-filled patches that penetrate your skin to numb nerve pain. Although some people report skin reactions, like a rash, others have found significant pain relief with the patches.

Capsaicin. This over-the-counter cream is made from hot red peppers. It sounds strange, but applying the hot pepper cream to your skin actually makes the area less sensitive to heat and pain. Wait until blisters have healed completely before using the cream. Keep in mind that capsaicin can cause allergic reactions in some people.

Your doctor can prescribe powerful pain medicine if you need it. Talk to her about your discomfort and speak up if any treatment is not working.

Ask around for shingles vaccine

Shingles comes with a blistering rash, but getting the vaccine can spare you those three to five weeks of discomfort. It is over 90 percent effective at preventing shingles and postherpetic neuralgia (PHN).

The CDC recommends that everyone over age 50 get both doses. You can even get it if you have already had shingles, to prevent another outbreak. However, researchers are still studying how long the vaccine will be effective.

Not all doctors' offices keep the shingles vaccine on hand. If yours doesn't, ask your pharmacist or local health clinic if they carry it. Remember to tell your doctor if you get vaccinated elsewhere, so she can note it in your file.

Dollars&Sense
4 steps to prescription safety

Even doctors and pharmacists make mistakes, and it's up to you to catch them. Keep prescription mistakes from killing you by following a few precautions.

Shop the same pharmacy. Have all your prescriptions filled at the same pharmacy. Each one tracks the medications you have filled there and checks for potential interactions — a safety check which could save your life.

Get to know your medications. Read the leaflets that come with your prescriptions. They contain important information about side effects, warnings, and drug interactions. If you have trouble understanding the leaflet, ask the pharmacist to go over it with you.

Do a double-check. Before you leave the pharmacy, open the bag and carefully read the label on each medication. Look for your name and check that the drug names, strengths, and dosage instructions match what your doctor told you. Ask the pharmacist to print your medicine labels in large type if you have trouble reading them.

Learn the lingo. You can decode your prescriptions with these common Rx abbreviations and their meanings.

Rx abbreviation	What it means	Rx abbreviation	What it means
a.c.	before meals	p.r.n.	as necessary
ad lib	as much as wanted	q.	every
b.i.d.	twice a day	q.4 h.	every four hours
h.	hour	q.d.	every day
h.s.	at bedtime	q.i.d.	four times a day
p.	after	q.o.d.	every other day
p.c.	after meals	Stat.	immediately
p.o.	by mouth	t.i.d.	three times a day

Sinusitis

Simple steps to unblock serious distress

Cold, allergy, or sinusitis? Many people have trouble telling the difference. They all produce similar symptoms — like a stuffy nose — but sinusitis is an inflammation that can develop into a serious infection. More than 37 million Americans share this misery and shell out $5.8 billion every year on sinus-related health care.

Acute sinusitis usually starts with a cold. If you treat it right, it may go away when the cold ends. Or it may develop into a painful infection and last a couple of weeks more, even after a trip to the doctor. With chronic sinusitis, sinus problems keep coming back or hang on for months at a time.

Whatever the extent of your sinusitis, you can get rid of some — if not all — of the suffering with a few simple practices. Most don't even cost much money. It's all about keeping your airways open, taking action that truly helps, and avoiding medicines that don't do any good.

Cheap and easy home solutions

Some of the best solutions to clogged sinuses are sitting right under your nose. And they don't require spending money at the drugstore for "miracle" sinus pills that may not give you relief.

Your sinuses are air-filled pockets located above and behind your eyes and nose. They have a lining that produces mucus to trap and carry away bacteria and irritants. When the sinuses swell, the mucus can't drain properly and it builds up, creating the perfect breeding ground for infection. That leads to more inflammation and swelling as well as painful pressure.

The trick is to drain those sinuses and get rid of the pressure and the mucus before it becomes infected. See how many of these time-tested home remedies will work for you.

Drink lots of water. Six or more glasses of water is the best way to lubricate your mucous membranes and keep them moist, so you can resist infection and your sinuses can drain easier. Experts say keeping hydrated may be the only treatment needed for mild sinusitis with no signs of infection.

Get the right rest. Not enough sleep can make your sinus problems more painful and longer lasting. Too much sleep can have the same effect. Help your sinuses drain at night by sleeping with your head slightly elevated. If one side is stuffier than the other, sleep with that side tilted down.

Breathe some steam. Fill the sink with hot water, put a towel over your head and the sink, and breathe in the warm vapors to get moisture into your sinuses. You can also hold a warm wet towel over your face, take a long steamy shower, or just breathe the steam from a cup of hot water or tea.

Try not to blow your nose when you have a cold. It forces mucus into your sinuses along with bacteria and viruses that can lead to sinusitis.

Wash out your nose. Rinsing nasal passages with salt water relieves congestion and other sinus problems. Researchers believe the salt helps break down mucus, but the main benefit is from the rinsing itself. Make your own wash with a quarter teaspoon table salt in 8 ounces of warm water. Use a bulb syringe to squirt this solution into one nostril and let it run out the other. Repeat with the other side, and after 30 seconds or so, gently blow out the remaining solution.

Spice up your food. Spicy foods and seasonings cut through sinus blockages. Eat more hot peppers, horseradish, and garlic. Use hot seasoning in soups and other dishes, and keep a bottle of hot sauce on the table.

Go for a brisk walk. Mild to vigorous exercise opens up nasal passages and clears breathing for many people. Others find it makes clogged sinuses worse. You need exercise anyway, so give it a try and see if it helps.

When sinus rinses do more harm than good

The very water you use to rinse your sinuses may actually be causing your sinus infections. Doctors sampled the germs living in the sinuses of people with chronic sinusitis, then sampled the tap water in their homes. Half had the same tough-to-kill bacteria in their sinuses as in their faucets, showers, and water filters. They had been rinsing their sinuses with water straight from those taps and filters.

Never use tap water as a sinus rinse, unless you boil it first for at least three minutes, then let it cool. Filters are no guarantee, either, since several people in this study had bacteria growing in their water filters. Use sterile water, available by prescription at your pharmacy. Or, if that's too expensive, buy distilled water at the store.

Smart tips for choosing OTCs

You can look to the drugstore for sinus relief, but choose over-the-counter remedies cautiously. It is easy to waste money on drugs that don't help, actually make your sinusitis worse, or have risky side effects.

It's important to know what causes your sinusitis so you can tailor treatment to your exact symptoms. Your doctor can help you figure that out. Then, stick to single-ingredient products instead of the drug combinations advertised as cold and sinus remedies so you won't load up on ingredients you don't need.

Use caution with decongestants. Decongestants may help your symptoms temporarily. They shrink your nasal passages, which promotes drainage. Unfortunately, they also thicken your mucus, making it more difficult to clear out your sinuses.

Inhaled decongestants have a dangerous rebound and dependency effect if you use them longer than three to five days. Oral decongestants can raise blood pressure and cause difficulty urinating. The Food and Drug Administration (FDA) has concluded that decongestants do not help with sinusitis and has ordered drug companies to take that information off their labels.

Steer clear of antihistamines. The only time they help sinusitis is when it's caused by allergies. Antihistamines dry out your sinuses and make your mucus more concentrated, which adds to inflammation and infection. And the older drugs that cause drowsiness intensify sinusitis fatigue.

Thin mucus with expectorants. These drugs generally cause mucus to be coughed up from the lungs and are sometimes recommended for sinusitis. They contain mucolytics — ingredients that thin mucous secretions — and help promote draining and reduce tissue swelling. Drink plenty of water to loosen mucus even further. Expectorants also may cause drowsiness or nausea.

Use standard pain relievers. If you suffer from mild fever and pain from sinus pressure, take your usual pain relievers like aspirin, acetaminophen, and ibuprofen. Remember that you will save money by buying the generic versions rather than brand names.

How to tell if it's sinusitis

	Sinusitis	Colds	Allergy
Common symptoms	nasal congestion, sore throat or coughing, facial pain or pressure		
Discharge	dark, thick, green, gray, or yellow mucus from nose or back of throat	runny nose with thin, clear-to-yellow mucus	runny nose with clear, watery mucus
Duration	acute, 1 to 3 weeks; chronic, 8 weeks or more	3 to 7 days	seasonal, lasts only when allergens are present
Other symptoms	fatigue, post-nasal drip	fatigue, sneezing	itchy eyes or nose

5 reasons to see the doctor

Sinusitis that turns into a sinus infection needs a doctor's attention. It's often hard to know when the viruses that cause colds and flu have given way to a bacterial infection you can stop with antibiotics. Signs you have progressed from a viral to a bacterial infection include:

▸ nasal congestion with a thick discharge that is yellowish to yellow-green or gray.

▸ facial or tooth pain, especially when you bend over.

▸ cold or flu symptoms that last 10 or more days.

- symptoms that worsen after five to seven days or return after initial improvement.

- high fever and sudden or severe illness.

Your doctor can decide if you need antibiotics, allergy medicine, or something else. If he thinks it is bacterial, he will probably give you an antibiotic that stops the most common bugs since the exact strain is difficult to determine. If you don't start improving in five or six days, you may need a different drug.

Replenish "good" bacteria wiped out by broad-spectrum antibiotics with *acidophilus* or *lactobacillus* found in live-culture yogurt.

You should take your medication at least 10 to 14 days and maybe as long as three weeks, even though you think you feel fine. Follow your doctor's instructions to the letter. If you stop the medicine too soon, you may not wipe out all the remaining bacteria. They will then continue to multiply and possibly become resistant to the antibiotic.

Top tips for healthy sinuses

Preventive measures can do as much to keep your sinuses healthy as steps you take to cure sinusitis.

Make wise food choices. The right diet helps heal and protect your mucous membranes and strengthen your immune system. Choose foods with lots of vitamins and minerals, particularly the ones below.

- **Vitamin C.** Fend off colds, allergies, and sinus infections with colorful fruits and vegetables like apricots, cantaloupe, strawberries, red and green peppers, kale, and broccoli.

- ▸ **Vitamin A.** Keep mucous membranes healthy with carrots, sweet potatoes, mangoes, and winter squash. They're full of beta carotene, which your body converts to vitamin A.

- ▸ **Zinc.** Strengthen your immunity with the zinc in beef liver, dark turkey meat, and black beans. It also helps change beta carotene to vitamin A.

Breathe the best air. Avoid cigarette smoke and other pollutants. If allergies fire up your sinus inflammation, take extra care to identify and avoid your particular allergens. Use a humidifier to put moisture back into the air, especially during dry winter months if you heat your home with a forced-air furnace. It makes it easier to breathe and keeps your sinuses from drying out.

Avoid pressure situations. Air travel can be difficult for sinusitis sufferers because of changes in pressure as the plane takes off and lands. Try decongestant nose drops or inhalers before a flight to avoid this problem.

Diving into a swimming pool isn't good for sinuses because it forces water up through your nasal passages. Chlorine in the pool irritates your nose and sinus lining. Drinking alcohol can also lead to sinus problems because it causes swelling in nasal and sinus membranes.

Brew sinus-soothing teas from your spice rack

When you're sick, there's nothing better than a hot cup of tea. The warm liquid soothes your throat and the steam can help break up congestion. But if you need a little extra relief, ditch the tea bags and take advantage of the remedies hidden in your pantry. These teas made from spices could be just what you need to soothe your sinusitis.

▸ Peppermint tea is a powerful, old-fashioned remedy for a stuffy nose. That's because peppermint leaves contain a compound called menthol. When you get a whiff, the vapors react with the cold receptors in your nose and make you feel like you're breathing in more cool air. This reduces that uncomfortable stuffed-up feeling and makes you feel as if you have taken a decongestant pill — even though you haven't.

To make a cup, add one to two tablespoons of fresh peppermint leaves or two to three teaspoons of dried peppermint leaves to a cup of freshly boiled water. Let this steep for 10 minutes, taking a few sniffs of the steam while you wait. Add sweetener, if needed, and slowly sip the tea while it works its magic on your poor nose. You may be surprised at how much better you feel.

▸ Fennel and anise both contain anti-inflammatory compounds that can help clear your sinuses. To make them into tea, crush one teaspoon of fennel seeds or one-and-a-half teaspoons of anise seeds with a mortar and pestle. Add to a cup of boiling water, and let steep for 10 to 15 minutes. Strain through a fine sieve or coffee filter, and enjoy.

▸ Sage tea is one great way to soothe a sore throat, so if you're dealing with a bad postnasal drip, give it a try. Add a teaspoon of ground sage to a cup of boiling water and let it steep for about 15 minutes.

Control your sweet tooth to fight sinusitis

Want to cripple your sinus defenses? Go ahead and eat that doughnut. Sweets are a surefire way to shift the balance of power to the bacterial invaders in your sinuses. Here's why you should step away from the sugar if you're prone to sinusitis.

Let your taste buds do their job. Your taste buds — and even other parts of your body like your upper airway and digestive tract — are armed with bitter and sweet taste receptors, though only those in your mouth send the taste sensation to your brain.

The bitter receptors are standing guard for your sinuses against bacteria and fungi that seek to do you harm.

When certain bacteria and fungi make their way into your airway, they give off a compound your bitter taste receptors may pick up. Your receptors then set off an alarm in your immune system. The message to fight the bad guys goes out within seconds to minutes.

Unfortunately, the sweet taste receptors don't see the world as a hostile place. They welcome bacteria and tell their bitter counterparts to sit back and relax. In other words, when you trigger your sweet taste receptors, you're telling those defensive bitter taste receptors to be quiet.

Relieve stuffy nasal passages with this simple addition to your vaporizer, recommended by the Vinegar Institute. Include 1/4 cup or more of vinegar in the amount of water the unit's instructions call for. Allow the vapor to fill the room. Breathe a sigh of sweet relief.

Don't excite your sweet tooth. The sweet taste receptors mean well. But what they're really doing when they get excited is allowing the bad guys past your built-in alarm system. Researchers already know that some bacteria use this to their advantage.

Staphylococcus aureus, which has been linked to sinusitis and other diseases caused by upper airway inflammation, is one such beast. Scientists discovered it can produce amino acids associated with sweetness at a concentration high enough to hold back your body's normal immune response to bitter taste receptors.

So what's a body to do? Well, researchers have already shown that eating lots of sugar may be linked to inflammatory stress and sinus symptoms. So pass on the sweet potato casserole and indulge in some oven-roasted Brussels sprouts instead. Your nose will thank you.

Sleep apnea

Say goodnight to bedtime breathing problems

British writer Anthony Burgess wrote, "Laugh and the world laughs with you; snore and you sleep alone." If you or your spouse snores, you know the truth in this saying. Loud snoring can be bothersome to those within earshot. It can also be a sign of sleep apnea, a dangerous condition estimated to affect 22 million people in America.

People with sleep apnea stop breathing during the night, from about 10 seconds to as long as a minute at a time. They awaken briefly to start breathing again, usually not realizing they have woken up. These incidents can happen hundreds of times each night.

Comic strips and television shows make fun of people who snore loudly, but sleep apnea is no joke. Recent research links sleep apnea to many serious health problems, including depression, strokes, heart attacks, high blood pressure, diabetes, and weight gain. It also makes you tired and cranky during the day, and it can lead to deadly traffic accidents.

Foolproof way to pin down your problem

Your doctor might send you for a sleep study, or polysomnograph, at a sleep center if he thinks you have sleep apnea. A sleep study can be expensive, easily costing $3,000 or more. Some insurance companies require a referral from your primary doctor. Some cover the cost of a study only if it's done in a sleep center accredited by the American Academy of Sleep Medicine.

What happens in a sleep study? Basically, you sleep overnight in a sleep center while your breathing, brain waves, muscle movement, and heart activity are monitored. You'll be hooked up to machines so sleep technicians can keep tabs on how you're doing and record your sleep. Follow these suggestions to make your sleep study as comfortable and productive as possible.

Pack your bags. Take your pajamas, toothbrush, clothes for the morning — the same things you need when you stay overnight in a hotel. A sleep center has individual sleeping rooms similar to hotel or hospital rooms, including facilities to shower in the morning. If you like a certain pillow or blanket, take it with you.

Watch what you drink. Avoid caffeine and alcohol before your sleep study, since they can change your sleep patterns and alter the test results.

> Don't take sleeping pills or tranquilizers if you have sleep apnea. These sleep aids can relax soft throat tissue, causing it to sag and making sleep apnea worse.

Prepare to get connected. Many sleep centers ask that you avoid using lots of hair gel, spray, or other products before a sleep study for easier attachment of electrodes and tapes to your head and scalp. Remove fingernail polish and artificial nails from at least two fingers. You'll wear a device called an oximeter on your finger to check your blood oxygen level through the nail. Also, avoid makeup, which can keep electrodes from sticking to the skin on your face.

Get there early. You'll be asked to arrive a couple hours before bedtime, since it takes about 45 minutes to connect leads, belts, and monitors, then more time for you to get relaxed for sleep.

Relax and enjoy the ride. Basically, the rest is up to you. Sleep as you normally do at home while the technicians and machines keep track of your sleep activities. Some people fear they won't be able to sleep connected to wires, but most people are so tired they have no trouble falling asleep.

For a list of accredited sleep disorders centers and laboratories for sleep-related breathing disorders in your area, check the American Academy of Sleep Medicine's Web site at *www.sleep education.org*.

Clever gadgets help you cope

How you treat your sleep apnea depends on the type of sleep apnea you have. Obstructive sleep apnea, caused when your tongue and throat muscles relax and block your airway, is the most common type. Central sleep apnea, when the brain doesn't send the right signal for breathing during sleep, is more common among people older than age 65. Complex sleep apnea is a combination of both types.

There's hope for people struggling to get a good night's sleep. Several gadgets can treat obstructive sleep apnea, helping you breathe and sleep better.

Mouth guards. For mild sleep apnea, doctors recommend you first try using a special dental appliance, similar to a sports mouth guard. These guards work by moving the jaw and tongue forward to allow for better breathing and less snoring. Your dentist should fit the guard to your mouth. Then, you should have a sleep study to be sure it's doing its job. Guards approved to treat sleep apnea are usually covered by health insurance.

Pillows. Specially made pillows that stretch the neck to improve air flow while you sleep work well for some people. Other pillows are designed to treat snoring and sleep apnea by encouraging you to sleep on your side.

Continuous positive airway pressure (CPAP). CPAP devices work by sending a constant stream of air through a mask over the nose and/or mouth to keep the airways open. This treatment works for about 80 to 90 percent of people, and it has the added benefit of lowering your blood pressure. But some people have trouble getting used to wearing a mask while sleeping, and it can cause side effects, like nasal congestion and dryness. In fact, one-third of those who try CPAP give it up. To increase your odds of success, see the following story *11 tips to make CPAP work for you*. CPAP machines can be rented or purchased, and they are usually covered by health insurance.

Disposable nasal valves. These stick to your nostrils like small, round bandages and create pressure when you exhale, which in turn keeps your airway open. How effective are they? Researchers have seen a 40 percent improvement in mild and moderate cases of sleep apnea. Each pair costs a couple of dollars, but you have to replace them each night. In addition, you'll need a doctor's prescription.

Sleep apnea linked to impotence

Men with sleep apnea are more likely to have impotence, also called erectile dysfunction (ED), or trouble getting or maintaining an erection. A recent study found that one commonly used treatment for impotence may only make things worse. In the study, men with severe sleep apnea took one dose of the drug Viagra, used to treat ED.

Researchers noted that the men had more incidents of interrupted breathing and lower oxygen levels in their blood as they slept — signs of worsened sleep apnea. The study was small, so more information is needed to know the full effects of Viagra on sleep apnea.

11 tips to make CPAP work for you

Using a continuous positive airway pressure (CPAP) device is the best way to treat obstructive sleep apnea, but it can be difficult to use. Give it your best shot, and try these hints from the American Academy of Sleep Medicine.

▸ **Start slowly.** Wear your CPAP for short periods during the day, perhaps while you relax or watch television.

▸ **Ramp up.** Use the setting that allows the machine to increase air pressure slowly.

▸ **Be consistent.** Use the CPAP every night and during naps. It works best if you sleep with it regularly. You'll get used to it sooner, too.

▸ **Muffle the noise.** Place the unit under your bed to dampen the sound if it keeps you awake. Newer CPAP models are nearly silent.

▸ **Adjust for fit.** The mask, headgear, tubing, and straps can be adjusted for the most comfort.

▸ **Ease congestion.** For mild nasal congestion, try a saline nasal spray. If you have serious congestion, ask your doctor if you should take a decongestant.

▸ **Dampen the air.** If you have trouble with breathing dry air, find a humidifier that fits your CPAP unit.

▸ **Try nasal pillows.** They add cushioning to the CPAP mask, making it more comfortable.

▸ **Keep it clean.** Once a week, clean the mask, tubing, and headgear.

▸ **Change the filter.** Check and replace the filters in the CPAP unit and humidifier regularly.

▸ **Ask for help.** Your doctor and machine supplier can make sure you have the correct machine, mask, and air pressure settings. Don't give up on CPAP without asking for help.

Latest news on surgical treatments

Surgery can treat sleep apnea, but it's not for everyone. Depending on how your mouth and throat are built and what is causing your sleep apnea, you may not be a good candidate. For many people, the problem can be solved through less-drastic measures, like losing weight or trying a CPAP machine.

Health insurance may not cover some surgical options, and they can be expensive. But for people with specific mouth or throat abnormalities, one of these procedures might be a good choice.

UPPP. Short for uvu-lopalatopharyngoplasty, UPPP is surgery to remove excess soft tissue at the back of the throat. If you still have tonsils or adenoids, they are also taken out. UPPP can expand your airway, allowing for better breathing at night, but the treatment isn't always successful. It's one of the most painful treatments, and recovery takes weeks. Common side effects include infection, voice changes, swallowing problems, changes in sense of smell, and excess mucus in the throat. Even worse, if you try UPPP and it doesn't work, using a CPAP machine can be less effective.

> Researchers found that wearing below-the-knee compression stockings only during the day reduced sleep apnea symptoms at night. The stockings help keep your blood circulating. This stops the buildup of fluid in your neck that contributes to snoring.

LAUP. This is a simpler version of UPPP that can be done in a doctor's office. Technically called laser-assisted uvulopalatoplasty, LAUP uses a laser to cut away the uvula, or tissue that hangs down at the back of the throat. It may take more than one session, and it's only good if the uvula is causing your trouble. This surgery also has low success rates, and it can cause throat dryness, narrowing, and scarring.

Radiofrequency ablation. Radio waves aimed at the base of the tongue heat, stiffen, and shrink small sections of tissue. It can be done in a doctor's office, requires about 10 treatments, and works best for mild sleep apnea.

Pillar implants. This reversible option shows promise, and it's less expensive and less painful than other surgical procedures. Braids of polyester are injected into the soft palate on the roof of the mouth, making it more rigid and less likely to collapse during sleep. Scar tissue forms around the braids to make them even stiffer.

Hypoglossal nerve stimulator. This surgically implanted device works like a pacemaker for sleep. An electrode in your chest senses when you start to inhale. Then another electrode, placed in your throat, stimulates your tongue to tighten, which keeps it from blocking your airway. A power source is inserted just below your collarbone. Doctors say this pacemaker improves symptoms by about 70 percent. But it's not recommended for people who are extremely overweight or who suffer from severe sleep apnea.

Get help from the experts

Kathleen, a 58-year-old research librarian, snored loudly and didn't sleep well for a year before her husband urged her to get help. Her doctor referred her for an overnight sleep study to determine if she had sleep apnea. Kathleen expected the worst when she agreed.

"My preconceived idea was that I would be sleeping on a cot in a lab," she recalls. "It was not at all like that." Instead, the sleep room was similar to a nice hospital room, with an adjoining bathroom, television, and simple furniture. And although she felt she didn't sleep well, she was successfully diagnosed with sleep apnea and fitted with a CPAP device to help her breathing. Now she's happy to be able to fall asleep quickly and get a good night's rest using the machine.

6 simple steps to more restful sleep

Not all people with sleep apnea snore, and not everyone who snores has sleep apnea. Snoring is quite widespread, affecting 57 percent of men and 40 percent of women in the United States. If you or your spouse snores on most nights, it's likely someone is longing for some peace and quiet.

People who may have sleep apnea should see a doctor for a diagnosis and treatment advice. You wouldn't want to merely quiet the snoring if it's a sign of a more serious health condition. But if snoring is your only problem, follow these steps to cut down on snoring and create a more peaceful bedroom.

> Playing the didgeridoo — that long, wooden, horn-like instrument from Australia — may reduce snoring and daytime sleepiness from sleep apnea. Researchers think regular practice strengthens muscles of the upper airway.

Lose excess weight. Here's another reason to pay more attention to your diet and exercise habits. Snoring is much more common among people who are overweight, probably because extra fat deposits in the throat make the airway narrower.

Stop smoking. If you avoid the nasal congestion that can come from smoking, you can probably also avoid the snoring it causes.

Avoid alcohol near bedtime. Alcohol narrows your breathing passages by relaxing the muscles in your airway, which leads to snoring. Although drinking alcohol may help you fall asleep faster, you'll wake up more during the night and have trouble falling back to sleep.

Sleep on your side. Sleeping on your back can cause your mouth to fall open and your throat to collapse, making snoring louder. If you have trouble staying on your side during the night, try sewing a pocket into the back of your pajamas and inserting a tennis ball. That'll send you back to your side.

Raise the head of your bed. One study found that sleeping in a more upright position could ease snoring. Raise yourself by propping up your back or head with pillows. You can also raise your bed by putting blocks of wood under your headboard.

Open your nasal passages. Some people only snore when they have a stuffy nose from colds or allergies. If that's you, try using the nasal strips many football players wear to breathe better. Studies show the strips reduce snoring in people with stuffy noses. Breathe Right is a well-known brand, but less-expensive, generic versions are also available.

What about the many other over-the-counter nasal sprays, drops, and remedies that promise to cure snoring? Research says these products claim to do a lot more good than they really do for most people. Don't waste your money.

Steer clear of drowsy driving accidents

Getting behind the wheel when you haven't had a good night's sleep is dangerous, yet more than half of all drivers have done it. No one plans to nod off while driving, but it's more likely to happen if you slept less than six hours the night before, or if you snore.

The National Sleep Foundation says you need to stop and rest if you experience blurry vision, trouble keeping your head up, yawning, or drifting from your lane.

Dollars&Sense
Medicine safety at home

Simple, clear instructions, with no confusing doctor-speak, on ways to take, store, and use medicines properly, can keep you safe from deadly drug interactions and accidental overdoses. Start with these tips for taking prescription drugs safely.

Focus on your task. Pay attention to what you are doing each time you take a pill, and you will be less likely to make mistakes.

▸ Keep medicines in their original bottles, unless placing them in pill boxes. Never store different drugs together in the same bottle.

▸ Take each medicine exactly as prescribed. Taking medicine too frequently in an effort to "speed up" the effects is a big mistake and can cause dangerous overdoses, even with seemingly harmless drugs like acetaminophen (Tylenol).

▸ Check with your pharmacist about the proper way to handle your meds. Not all pills can safely be crushed, dissolved, or split.

▸ Mark the lids and labels of your medicines with different colored stickers or nail polishes to help tell them apart.

▸ Read the label every time you take a medicine to make sure you are taking the right one, the right way.

▸ Turn on the light when you take medicines at night to be sure you get the right ones. Read the label under bright light. Your eyes need about three times more light to read at age 60 than they did at age 30.

▸ Don't take anyone else's drugs. They can mask important symptoms from your doctor and interact dangerously with other medications.

▸ Continue taking a medicine for as long as your doctor tells you to, even if you start feeling better. Always talk to your doctor before you stop taking a drug.

Store them properly. Store medications in a cool, dry, dark place like a kitchen cabinet or bedroom shelf. Don't keep them in the bathroom, where heat and moisture can damage them, and don't store them in the refrigerator unless your doctor, pharmacist, or the drug's label says to do so.

Toss out the old. Clean out your medicine cabinet every six months and toss expired over-the-counter (OTC) and prescription drugs. Old medications are not only unsafe, but they probably won't work. Don't flush them down the toilet, however. Drugs leach into the water supply, contaminating streams, fish, and eventually people. Instead, ask your pharmacy or doctor's office to dispose of them.

Never forget another dose. Remembering to take all your medicines is no small challenge, especially if you have complicated dosing schedules. Try this advice to stay on track.

▸ Plan ahead by organizing pills in a pillbox.

▸ Tape notes strategically around the house on the bathroom mirror, by the coffee pot, on the bedside clock, and elsewhere to remind you to take your meds.

▸ Establish a buddy system with a friend who also takes pills daily. Take turns calling each other when it's time for the next dose.

▸ Use a small chalkboard or dry erase board to stay on track. Put a check mark and the time next to each drug name when you take it. Erase them all the next day and start over.

Get an annual Rx check-up. Once a year, bring all your medications to the doctor's office for a "medicine check-up" — including all prescriptions, OTC drugs, supplements, vitamins, and herbal remedies you use regularly. Have him go over the dosage instructions, warnings, and possible interactions with you, and ask if you can stop taking any of them.

Fill him in on OTCs. Let your doctor know if you use OTC remedies regularly. Most are not meant for long-term use, and your doctor may be able to prescribe a more effective medication.

Stroke

Best ways to thwart a brain attack

Every 40 seconds someone in the United States has a stroke. Stroke, also called brain attack, ranks third behind heart disease and cancer as a cause of death.

Ischemic stroke, the most common type, occurs when a blood clot blocks blood vessels to the brain, or in the brain, cutting off the brain's supply of oxygen. In a hemorrhagic stroke, a blood vessel bursts, leading to bleeding in or around the brain. Both types of stroke can have devastating results. Besides killing you, stroke can also affect your motor skills, speech, memory, behavior, senses, and thought processes depending on which parts of your brain are damaged.

Who does stroke target? Black people, seniors, men, and those with a family history of stroke are at higher risk. Other risk factors include high blood pressure, high cholesterol, heart disease, diabetes, smoking, and obesity. Luckily, you can protect yourself from a brain attack. Discover what steps you can take to prevent, recognize, and recover from a stroke.

Save a life with swift action

Every second counts when it comes to a stroke. The longer oxygen remains cut off from your brain, the more damage occurs.

Often, acting quickly can be the difference between life and death. That's why it's so important to know the symptoms of a stroke and how to respond to a brain attack.

Recognize the signs. Symptoms of a stroke include sudden weakness or numbness of the face, arm, or leg, especially on one side of the body; confusion; trouble speaking or understanding; difficulty seeing; dizziness, loss of balance or coordination; and a sudden, severe headache.

Even if the symptoms pass quickly without any lasting effects, don't ignore them. They could be warning signs of a transient ischemic attack, or TIA. These "mini-strokes" often come before a full-blown stroke, and they should be taken seriously.

Give a pop quiz. When you suspect someone is having a stroke, ask the person these three simple questions:

You definitely grow older on your birthday. But, according to a recent study, you are also 27 percent more likely to have a stroke, TIA, or heart attack. The added stress could be to blame.

▶ Can you smile?

▶ Can you raise both arms above your head?

▶ Can you speak a complete sentence?

If the person has trouble with any of these tasks, take immediate action.

Call for help. If you think you — or someone else — may be having a stroke, call 911 right away. You can also drive the person to the hospital. But never let someone having a stroke drive himself — and never attempt to drive yourself if you are the one experiencing the stroke.

2 ways to prevent a second stroke

Once you've had a stroke, you increase your risk of having another one. That's where blood thinners come in. Antiplatelet drugs, like aspirin, and anticoagulants, like warfarin, help prevent blood clots from forming. Your doctor may suggest these drugs if you are at high risk for stroke, if you've had a transient ischemic attack (TIA), or to prevent a second stroke.

Antiplatelets. Aspirin and other antiplatelet drugs, keep the platelets in your blood from clumping together. Aspirin, the most common antiplatelet drug, can lower your risk of a second stroke.

During a stroke, it's as if your brain ages in dog years — 8.7 hours every second, 3.1 weeks every minute, 3.6 years every hour, and a whopping 36 years for an untreated stroke.

Anticoagulants. These drugs thin your blood and prevent it from clotting. The most common anticoagulant is warfarin (Coumadin), which is often prescribed to people with multiple risk factors for stroke.

However, blood-thinning drugs come with risks. Because they prevent your blood from clotting, they may increase your risk of bleeding. While they protect against ischemic stroke, they slightly increase your risk for hemorrhagic stroke.

When taking these common prescription drugs, you should never consume too much vitamin K. This vitamin, found in broccoli, spinach, cabbage, kale, and brussels sprouts, makes warfarin less effective, which increases your risk of blood clots. This is critical news you probably haven't heard from your doctor or pharmacist. Several drugs and supplements can also interfere with warfarin, so make sure to tell your doctor about any medication you are taking.

Similarly, the FDA recently issued a warning about the danger of taking ibuprofen with aspirin. Mixing these two painkillers can lessen the antiplatelet effect of aspirin.

'Plane' truth about blood clots

Your next flight may leave you with more than just jet lag. Flying increases your risk of deep vein thrombosis, or painful blood clots in your legs. That may have something to do with the low cabin pressure during flights or just sitting still for so long. Deep vein thrombosis is a common complication following a stroke because of the stroke victim's limited mobility.

No matter what the reason for the risk, you can take steps to lessen it. On long flights, get up and stretch your legs often. Drink plenty of water to stay hydrated, and avoid alcoholic beverages and sleeping pills. Compression stockings may also help. You can find them for as little as $16, but a good pair will cost about $60.

Simple strategies for stroke prevention

Experts estimate that more than half of all strokes could be prevented. Here are some terrific tactics to sidestep stroke.

- **Control high blood pressure.** High blood pressure, the No. 1 risk factor for stroke, contributes to 54 percent of all strokes. Keep your blood pressure within a healthy range. For helpful tips on how to do that, check out the *High blood pressure* chapter.

- **Quit smoking.** Smokers have a greater risk of stroke than nonsmokers. Cigarettes boost your risk of both ischemic and hemorrhagic stroke. You should also do your best to avoid secondhand smoke.

- **Lose weight.** Obesity, especially abdominal obesity, dramatically boosts your risk of stroke. Cut back on calories and become more active to shed those extra pounds.

- **Exercise regularly.** Being a couch potato can triple your risk of stroke compared to people who are physically active. Exercise helps you overcome stroke risk factors like obesity and high blood pressure. Aim for at least 30 minutes of activity a day.

- **Avoid alcohol.** Drinking moderately may reduce your risk of ischemic stroke, but it boosts your risk of hemorrhagic stroke. Heavy drinking causes several health problems, like raising your blood pressure and producing irregular heartbeats, that can increase your stroke risk. Limit yourself to no more than two drinks a day.

- **Improve your cholesterol.** Boosting your HDL, or good, cholesterol can reduce your risk of stroke. So can lowering your total and LDL, or bad, cholesterol. Eat a healthy diet, exercise, and take cholesterol-lowering medication, if necessary, to achieve your goals.

Negative emotions, such as anger, fear, irritability, or nervousness, may also contribute to stroke. Find ways to stay calm or avoid stressful situations. Air pollution may also boost your risk of ischemic stroke, so moving from the city to the country might do you some good.

You may need nine hours of sleep to feel bright-eyed and bushy-tailed when your partner feels wide awake after just six. Everyone's sleep needs vary, but research suggests between six and eight hours each night is the sweet spot for stroke protection. Consistently getting more or less shut-eye could put you at a greater risk.

Foil stroke with healthy foods

What you put in your belly can help safeguard your brain. To ward off stroke, make sure your menu includes plenty of the following foods.

Fruits and veggies. Several studies have found that eating more fruits and vegetables reduces your risk of stroke. In fact, a recent British study determined that eating three to five servings of fruits and vegetables each day lowers your stroke risk by 11 percent. If you eat more than five servings, you've slashed your stroke risk by 26 percent. Here's why — fruits and veggies are loaded with potassium, folate, fiber, and antioxidants like vitamin C, beta carotene, and flavonoids.

Orange juice. Why take Bayer when you can eliminate blood clots with a juicy, natural "formula" that won't upset your stomach? Rich in vitamin C, which has been shown to reduce the risk of stroke, oranges also contain more than 60 flavonoids. Many of these antioxidants have the power to stop blood clots from forming. Other fruit juices, like grape or cranberry, can also help. One glass a day should do the trick.

Spinach. Popeye's favorite veggie, a great source of the B vitamin folate, has protected against stroke in both human and animal studies. Other good sources of folate include legumes, peas, asparagus, and enriched breads, cereals, and pastas.

Fish. Fatty fish contain omega-3 fatty acids, which help with stroke risks like high blood pressure, high cholesterol, and inflammation. But how you prepare your fish makes a difference. A recent Harvard study found that eating tuna or other baked or broiled fish lowers your risk of stroke, but munching on fried fish and fish sandwiches actually increases your risk.

Whole grains. The fiber in whole grains fights both high blood pressure and high cholesterol, making it an ideal weapon against stroke. Cereal fiber, the kind in oats, wheat, rye, and barley, provides the most protection.

Dairy foods. A recent study found that calcium may lessen the severity of a stroke and improve your chances of recovery. Besides low-fat dairy products, good sources of calcium include legumes, green vegetables like broccoli and kale, and canned fish with bones, like sardines.

Your diet should also include plenty of potassium and magnesium, two more minerals that help regulate blood pressure and guard against stroke. Bananas, dried fruits, molasses, cereals, nuts, and raw vegetables provide potassium, while you can find magnesium in seafood, dry beans, whole grains, and nuts.

Sweet to arteries, bitter toward plaque: How dark chocolate stacks up to stroke

Laughter may be the best medicine, but sometimes you need a dose of chocolate — so goes a popular saying. Historians think that decadent bite of ground cocoa beans has tempted people as far back as 4,000 years, and it continues to impress with health benefits today. Indulge in one of these treats every day and you could reduce your risk of stroke and open up your artery walls.

Chocolate contains flavanols like epicatechin, catechin, and procyanidins that favor your heart. Science says they may interrupt inflammation, lower blood pressure, and fend off clots that close off your arteries.

In a recent meta-analysis of 14 studies involving 508,705 people, researchers concluded that eating one to six servings of chocolate a week may be ideal for reducing the risk of stroke.

It's not just the Beach Boys who feel good vibrations. Vibrating insoles may improve your balance after a stroke, according to Boston University researchers.

In another review, stroke risk dropped 21 percent for those who ate the most chocolate compared to those who ate the least. But that's no excuse to scarf down the candy aisle, say researchers. Eating more than 100 grams a week — the amount found in two chocolate snack bars — delivers enough calories, sugar, and fat to cancel out the benefits.

Make a smart choice for a smaller serving of about an ounce of dark chocolate. That's about the size of a pack of dental floss. Look for the kind with at least 70 percent to 85 percent cocoa to get the most flavanols.

Smog and smoke — new risk for stroke

Sound the alarm. A shocking source has just been ranked one of the top 10 causes of stroke.

Scientists already know air pollution is linked to damage in your lungs, heart, and brain. But they were surprised to learn about a third of strokes can be chalked up to impure air.

They suspect toxins that breeze about big cities cause inflammation and oxidative stress. These two terrors trigger changes in your arteries and raise blood pressure.

"People should limit their exposure on days with higher air pollution levels," says scientist Tao Liu, Ph.D., "especially those with high blood pressure."

Check *AirNow.gov* to find out the quality of your outdoor air. And remember, it's not all about outside. Cooking fumes, fireplace smoke, and chemicals can contribute to bad air quality. To clear the air under your roof, try an air purifier, run an exhaust fan in your bathroom and kitchen, and replace old wood stoves.

Urinary tract infections

Head off problems before they start

Bad bacteria sometimes multiply in the urethra, kidneys, or bladder, resulting in a urinary tract infection (UTI). As many as 1 in 2 women have a UTI in their lifetime compared to about 1 in 10 men. Diabetes, kidney stones, and an enlarged prostate also up the risk, as does wearing a catheter.

While some people experience classic UTI symptoms — a frequent urge to urinate, burning, and cloudy or reddish urine — seniors may not. Instead, they may experience nausea, vomiting, abdominal pain, confusion, coughing, or shortness of breath.

Seeing a doctor for diagnosis is important. Although most urinary tract infections are mild and easily treated, they can lead to kidney stones, kidney scarring, and, in postmenopausal women, incontinence.

You'll probably need a course of antibiotics to kick a UTI, but the easiest remedy is to prevent infection in the first place. Start with these natural home remedies to help urinary problems, all without drugs or surgery.

'Berry' the burn of UTIs

Long before antibiotics, cranberries reigned as a popular remedy for urinary tract infections (UTIs). Science proves they still do.

Drinking cranberry juice daily can prevent UTIs and curb the need for expensive antibiotics and doctor visits.

The red pigments, or proanthocyanidins, in cranberries and blueberries seem to keep UTI-causing bacteria from clinging to the walls of your urinary tract. Without a good grip, bacteria such as *E. coli* can't dig in and cause infection. Cranberry juice, in particular, seems to keep regular bacteria as well as antibiotic-resistant super bugs from getting a foothold in the urinary tract.

But these berries work best as preventive measures, not treatments for existing infections. Some evidence suggests sexually active adult women could see a 50-percent drop in recurring UTIs with cranberry juice or supplements. However, no solid evidence shows the fruit can cure existing infections.

Experts suggest anywhere from 8 ounces of 100-percent pure, unsweetened cranberry juice daily, to 8 to 16 ounces of cranberry juice cocktail a day. If you prefer supplements, try taking one 300- to 400-milligram cranberry tablet twice daily. It may take four to eight weeks to see results.

People prone to oxalate kidney stones should talk to their doctor before starting cranberry therapy, as long-term use could raise the risk of these stones. Also, discuss it with your doctor if you take the blood thinner warfarin (Coumadin), as the berries could boost its effect.

Say good-bye to urinary problems

Simply adding a few common foods to your diet could spell the end of urinary tract infections. What could be easier? Experts believe some foods help keep bacteria from invading the urinary tract.

Cool the burn with creamy treat. Most UTIs are caused by bad bacteria from stool contaminating the urethra. In premenopausal women, the vagina is home to *lactobacilli*, a family of good bacteria that includes acidophilus. *Lactobacilli* create an unfriendly environment for bad bugs such as *E. coli*, the main cause of uncomplicated UTIs. *Lactobacilli* levels naturally drop after menopause, perhaps one reason older women are prone to UTIs. Adding back the good bugs through diet could help reverse that trend.

A Finnish study involving more than 200 premenopausal women found those who ate fermented dairy products like yogurt and cheese at least three times a week were almost 80 percent less likely to develop a UTI as women who ate them less than once a week. Fresh dairy such as milk had no protective effect. Other studies show taking probiotics supplements helps restore the natural balance of bacteria in the urinary and genital areas.

Move over, cranberries. This same Finnish study delivered more good news. Along with cranberries, eating fresh strawberries, raspberries, cloudberries, lingonberries (a European relative of cranberries), or drinking juices made from these berries all lowered women's risk for UTIs. Researchers say you can thank flavonols, natural compounds plants make to ward off their own microbial infections. Fruits such as apples, plums, and cherries are packed with flavonols, but in general berries boast the highest amounts.

> Over-the-counter remedies such as AZO Urinary Pain Relief can temporarily ease UTI symptoms like burning and itching, but they will not cure the underlying infection.

Find big relief with tiny seeds. Grapefruit seeds seem to have antibacterial powers that could be used to treat urinary tract infections. Four case studies from Nigeria found eating five to six grapefruit seeds every eight hours for two weeks cleared up urinary tract infections without the need for antibiotics. In one man's case, the seeds even seem to have worked against antibiotic-resistant bacteria. Research has confirmed that grapefruit seed extract has the same antimicrobial properties. Get your doctor's advice on this remedy before trying it. Remember, UTIs can become serious if not treated properly.

Clean up your act for a healthy tract

How you handle matters "down there" has a lot to do with whether or not you get urinary tract infections. Practicing a few hygiene tips could help slash your incidence of UTIs.

▸ Wipe front to back after using the restroom. Wash urinary and genital areas with soapy water or wet wipes after each bowel movement.

▸ Urinate both before and after sex to empty the bladder and flush bacteria from the urethra.

▸ Wear underwear and stockings with cotton crotches, and change them at least once a day. Avoid wearing tight pants.

▸ Avoid using bath oils, feminine hygiene sprays, powders, or any other perfumed products near the genital area, especially if you have skin allergies.

A little less than half of women with UTI-like symptoms actually have a different condition such as vaginitis, interstitial cystitis, or irritation of the urethra.

▸ Use sanitary napkins rather than tampons, and change them after each urination. Some experts think tampons encourage the development of UTIs.

▸ Take showers instead of baths. Soaking in a tub helps bacteria enter the urethra.

Prevent catheter-associated UTIs

Catheters cause about three out of four of the UTIs people get in hospitals. The longer you wear a catheter, the higher your risk of infection. Having diarrhea while wearing a catheter pushes that risk even higher.

Whether you need a catheter for a few days or few months, you can take steps to protect yourself from bacterial infection.

▸ Remember to drink plenty of fluids, and aim for three glasses of cranberry juice daily.

- Wash your hands before touching the catheter or the area around it.

- Clean the catheter and the surrounding area gently with soap and water daily and after each bowel movement.

- Keep the catheter tube free of kinks and knots.

- Stabilize the drainage bag against your leg using tape or bandages. Be careful not to wrap them so tight you cut off blood flow in the leg.

- Keep the drainage bag off the floor.

2 healthy ways to drown bad bacteria

Never underestimate a UTI. Left untreated, the infection can spread to your kidneys and cause permanent damage. The key to protecting yourself may be in what you drink.

With water you don't need to wish you're well. Do you limit how much you drink just to avoid frequent bathroom trips? Well, stop. You can get an infection if bad bacteria enter your urinary tract through the urethra and multiply. And a great way to keep this bacteria at bay is — you guessed it — to flush it out by drinking water.

A study in *JAMA Internal Medicine* followed 140 premenopausal women with frequent cystitis — a bladder inflammation often caused by a UTI. Researchers found that women prone to cystitis episodes halved the number of recurrences when they drank an extra 6 cups of water each day for a year.

Urinary and respiratory infections cause confusion, fever, and dizziness — all symptoms that could knock you off your feet. In fact, infections factor into 45 percent of falls. Be on the lookout for early warning signs like weakness or fatigue, and be sure to tell your doctor.

Green tea battles bad bacteria. "Thank God for tea!" wrote Sydney Smith, preacher and founder of the prestigious British periodical *The Edinburgh Review*. "What would the world do without tea! How did it exist?" Fortunately, you don't have to imagine a world without tea — which is good news if you suffer from UTIs.

Natural compounds in green tea are known to fight bad bacteria. So researchers at Oakland University William Beaumont School of Medicine examined the effects of green tea extract on UTI-causing bacteria — specifically *E.coli*. They found the polyphenols in green tea, especially epicatechin-3-gallate (ECG), kept the bacteria from growing.

Drinking just 1 cup of green tea could positively affect the bacteria in your urinary tract, and several cups throughout the day could provide long-lasting protection.

The wonder herb that fights off infection

Good news for garlic lovers everywhere — this flavor-enhancing food may help your bladder, too.

Allicin is a compound produced when you chop or crush garlic. It doesn't just give garlic its characteristically pungent smell. Along with other sulfur compounds, it's the force behind garlic's antimicrobial punch. In fact, garlic's effect even holds up against bacteria that has become drug-resistant.

In a study out of India's Birla Institute of Technology and Sciences, garlic extract faced off against 166 bacteria strains isolated from the urine of people with urinary tract infections. Scientists found that over 80 percent of the antibiotic-resistant bacteria they tested was impacted by the garlic.

Although this is still early research, garlic may turn out to be one spicy way to fight UTIs.

Dollars&Sense
Spot the truth behind health claims

New treatments spring up every day promising to cure whatever ails you. Scam artists tend to target people with chronic or incurable conditions like arthritis, obesity, memory loss, Alzheimer's disease, cancer, or diabetes. Don't get taken for a ride.

Proven treatments undergo years of study before experts start recommending them. Look at the evidence backing a remedy, and consider these questions.

▸ Who funded the research? Did the company selling the product pay for the studies or did a nonbiased group like the National Institutes of Health?

▸ Was the study done with people, animals, or test tubes? Results from animal and lab experiments don't mean a treatment will work in people.

▸ If the trial involved people, did it meet the "gold standard?" That is, was it randomized, double-blinded, and placebo-controlled?

▸ How many people took part in the study, and for how long? In general, the more people tested and the longer a study lasts, the more meaningful the results.

One place to find easy-to-read, unbiased information about herbs, nutrition, and alternative supplements is the Office of Dietary Supplements, a department of the National Institutes of Health. Visit the Web site *ods.od.nih.gov,* and click on "Health Information."

The Food and Drug Administration (FDA) issues warnings and recalls via a toll-free information line at 888-463-6332 and on its Web site at *www.fda.gov/safety/recalls-market-withdrawals-safety-alerts*. You can also use the site to sign up to receive email alerts about recalls, market withdrawals, and safety information.

Weight gain
Proven solutions for a serious problem

More than 1.9 billion people in the world are either obese or overweight, and the numbers are expanding rapidly. Excess weight boosts your risk of serious diseases like type 2 diabetes, heart disease, stroke, and some forms of cancer. Obesity costs Americans more than $150 billion every year in medical costs and lost productivity.

Weight gain is not a mystery. When you put more fuel — or food — into your body than you burn, the excess energy is stored as fat. To manage your weight, you must balance intake with output.

The search is always on for a quick and easy solution — a miracle diet, magic pill, or super exercise machine. But in the end, the only proven solution is a combination of sensible eating habits and regular exercise.

7 no-nonsense ways to shed extra pounds

Without making a few lifestyle changes, you'll always have a hard time maintaining a healthy weight. Here are some tips to help you.

Practice portion control. Researchers at Cornell University discovered something interesting while hosting an ice cream social. When people serve themselves, they tend to put more food on their plates if the plates and serving utensils are large. Think small and cut back on the size of your helpings by using smaller plates, bowls, and serving utensils. And when you're eating out, don't fall for the fast food "supersize" craze.

Pound the pillow. Women who sleep only five or six hours a night gain more weight than those who get seven hours of sleep a night, according to the Nurses' Health Study. Another study found that two key hormones that regulate appetite get out of whack when you don't get enough sleep. Leptin, which tells your body you've eaten enough, decreases, and ghrelin, which stimulates your appetite, increases.

Turn off the TV. Your risk for obesity increases 23 percent for every two hours a day you spend in front of your TV. Americans now burn 111 fewer calories a day than in years past, and that adds up to 11 pounds a year. When you're sitting around watching TV, not only does your metabolism slow, you might be tempted by clever advertisers to reach for high-sugar, high-fat snacks — and empty calories.

> Many so-called "healthy foods" are actually loaded with sugar and fat. Read the nutritional labels when you replace junk food with yogurt, granola, and low-fat snacks.

Volunteer your services. Retirees who joined a program to help mentor and tutor children in local elementary schools more than doubled their physical activity, a Johns Hopkins University survey shows. Not only did the volunteers get off the couch and away from the TV, they had more energy for daily activities like household chores and gardening.

Find strength in numbers. You can lose more weight by joining an organized weight loss group than trying to go it alone, says a study funded by the U.S. Department of Agriculture. Women dieting on their own have higher stress levels, and that leads to less success overall. A group also gives you support and nutritional information you won't get by yourself.

Don't use food as a crutch. When you eat to cope with anger, depression, or stress, you're loading up on food that makes you fat. Find something else to help you deal with your emotions — go for a walk, take a relaxing bath, or play a game.

Forget about skipping meals. Eating three meals a day and a healthful snack or two keeps your blood sugar stable and your hunger pangs under control. In addition, missing a meal can encourage you to overeat at the next meal. Overeating stretches your stomach, which continues to signal hunger until it gets back to normal size.

Win the fat war

It's easy to find a diet plan that will knock off several pounds fairly quickly, but the trick is keeping off those pounds for good. In a recent study, researchers concluded it doesn't make much difference which diet plan you use as long as you stick with it.

The study results showed weight loss was about the same for the Atkins, Ornish, Weight Watchers, and the Zone diet plans. Unfortunately, only 50 to 65 percent of the participants stayed with their diets for the full year of the study. Here's a look at some of the most popular diet plans.

▸ **Restricted calories.** The more you cut calories, the faster you'll lose weight. But watch out for cutting back too much. Extreme diets of less than 1,100 calories can have serious health consequences, and you're more likely to binge or overeat when you go off the diet.

▸ **High protein, low carbohydrate.** These diets are proving to be effective for short-term weight loss, but experts are concerned about their long-term effects on your health. The Atkins diet emphasizes high-protein and low-carbohydrate intake, while the South Beach and the Zone diets allow certain types of carbs.

▸ **Low fat, high-fiber.** This approach is to replace fat with complex carbohydrates, like fruits, vegetables, and whole grains. You count grams of fat instead of calories. But when you eliminate fat, you may miss out on some important nutrients. Commercial "low-fat" products are also likely to be loaded with sugar and other ingredients with no nutritional value.

The simplest and least expensive weight loss plan is to cut back on calories and exercise for at least 30 minutes a day, five times a week. Cutting fat, protein, or carbohydrates may make a diet fashionable or easy to follow, but it only works when you burn more calories than you take in. Depending on your age, gender, and activity level, you need 12 to 15 calories a day per pound of your desired weight.

The best way for you to lose weight — and keep it off — is to find a plan you'll stick with. It should give you proper nutrition, yet allow you to control your calories. You could also rely more on making healthy food choices rather than following a strict diet. No matter what plan you choose, make sure you find time to exercise.

Simple secret makes losing weight easier

Eating breakfast helps you lose weight — and keep it off. Nearly four out of five people in the National Weight Control Registry, a survey of almost 3,000 people who have lost at least 30 pounds and kept it off for a year or more, eat breakfast every day.

The right kind of breakfast keeps you from getting hungry and loading up on calories later in the day. Choose whole grain cereals and fruit, but steer clear of sugary cereals. Sugar, a simple carbohydrate, raises your blood sugar quickly — then it falls, and you're hungry again. Both whole grains and eggs, another breakfast favorite, will help you feel full longer.

Order up veggies to stem weight gain

Imagine you had the chance to invite singer Paul McCartney and boxer Mike Tyson over for dinner. What a night that would be. But what would you serve them?

Seems like such different men would have very different tastes indeed. But if truth be told, your guests would probably pick tofu and quinoa over a grilled T-bone. Why? Because they understand the benefits of a vegetarian diet.

So how could retreating from meat help you? A study recently published in the journal *Nutrients* gives some insight.

Sidestep the spare tire by going vegetarian. The 10-year Spanish study of 16,000 university graduates found that those who ate a vegetarian diet were less likely to become obese as years passed compared to folks who favored meatier meals.

At the start of the study, participants filled out detailed food questionnaires that awarded them points according to the amount of plant foods — fruits, vegetables, grains, legumes, olive oil, and nuts — they ate each day. Points were taken off for animal fats, dairy, eggs, fish, seafood, and meat. The participants were then divided into five groups based on their total scores.

At the end of the study, the researchers discovered that people with the most pro-vegetarian diets were 43 percent less likely to become obese compared to those who ate the most animal foods.

Why do plant-eaters tend to be slimmer? Experts believe they've gotten to the root of the matter. For one, all the fiber and phytochemicals found in fruits and veggies are kind to your waistline, while the high-calorie saturated fat found in meat is not.

In addition, some doctors think vegetarians may pay more attention to other areas of their health, not just their diet. For instance, they may exercise more and smoke less.

The authors of the Spanish study boiled their findings down to this. "Plant-based diets are associated with substantially lower risk of developing obesity. This supports current recommendations to shift to diets rich in plant foods, with lower intake of animal foods."

Couple healthier living with healthier eating, and you're one step closer to hanging on to that slim, trim figure for life.

'Light' drinks: Weight loss wonder or diet blunder?

Enjoy that mid-afternoon Snickers bar with a low-calorie diet soda instead of a regular soft drink, and you will cut calories. But you may be sabotaging your weight loss plan.

Researchers from Johns Hopkins University studied diet beverages and calorie consumption in adults. Here's what they found.

▸ Among overweight and obese adults, diet beverage drinkers took in more calories from food than people who drank sugar-sweetened beverages. The researchers suspect they may eat extra food to make up for the missing calories. Artificial sweeteners might also increase your appetite or affect the "sweet sensors" in your brain, decreasing the satisfaction you get from eating something sweet. If you want to use diet drinks to lose weight, the study authors suggest you track how many calories you eat and drink, and make sure you're reducing your total calorie intake.

▸ Among people who weren't overweight or obese, diet beverage drinkers took in fewer total calories a day than people who drank sugar-sweetened beverages. So if your weight is normal, switching from sugar-sweetened beverages to diet drinks may help you prevent weight gain.

That's why some experts suggest you limit or eliminate both sugar-sweetened beverages and diet drinks. Instead, emphasize better choices like water, sparkling water, and unsweetened coffee or tea.

Slim down with water

Here's a weight-loss stunner. Researchers found that drinking just 4 ounces of H2O, 20 minutes before meals, stimulates weight loss — even if you do nothing else. And a study of more than 18,000 adults showed that people who drank one to three cups of plain, ordinary water daily knocked up to 200 calories off their total intake.

Experts think some of the extra calories burn up as your body heats the water. But all that water makes you feel fuller, too, and that helps you eat less.

Your restaurant survival guide: 13 tips for guilt-free dining

Eating out adds 200 extra calories to your daily total, reports a study in *Public Health Nutrition*. You'd get nearly the same number from downing an entire Hershey's Milk Chocolate Bar. But no, you don't have to stop dining out. Just use some clever tricks to find low-calorie items hidden in the restaurant menu.

▶ Call ahead or check the restaurant's nutrition information on its Web site to find healthy, low-calorie dishes. Before you try to guess calories by looking at the dish or its menu description, consider this. A survey of over 3,000 adults and youngsters found that people underestimated the calorie content of restaurant food by at least 175 calories — and some missed it by a whopping 500 calories. The higher the calories in a meal, the more people misjudged. If you can't actually check calories, order from the low-calorie or heart-healthy menu, or ask your server which low-calorie dishes are the healthiest.

▸ Order water, unsweetened tea, fat-free or low-fat milk, or other drinks without added sugars.

▸ Ask for whole-wheat bread or a wrap if you order a sandwich.

▸ Avoid the all-you-can-eat buffet. Order off the menu instead.

▸ Beware the super-size bargain. Think twice before you upgrade to the larger portion for a lower price per serving. It may be a good deal, but you'll get too many calories if you eat it all at once. Only consider upgrades like these if you share with another person or take home the extra food for another meal. Sharing and doggy bags are also a good way to keep from eating regular-size portions that are too high in calories.

▸ Ask for salad dressing on the side so you can choose how much to use. Watch out for salad saboteurs including high-fat dressings, candied nuts, and meats that are breaded or drowning in sauce. Also, avoid salads where the vegetables and fruit are outnumbered by meats, cheeses, mayo, croutons, and other ingredients high in saturated fats or calories.

▸ Choose main dishes that include vegetables and grains, such as stir-fries, red beans and rice, kebobs, or pasta with a tomato sauce.

▸ Avoid fried dishes, ordering options that are grilled, broiled, or steamed instead.

▸ Opt for the small, medium, or appetizer size if the entree, drink, or side dish comes in more than one size.

▸ Order all sauces on the side.

- Ask for substitutions. For example, switch out a side of fries for rice pilaf, or Alfredo sauce for marinara.

- Never add butter or salt to foods.

- Enjoy fresh fruit for dessert.

Foolproof way to burn fat and build muscle

Exercise is a double-barreled weapon in the fight against weight gain. It not only helps you burn more calories, it builds muscle, which burns calories faster than fat tissue. On top of that — people who exercise are more likely to stick to a weight loss plan.

Here's more good news. Taking a brisk walk might help you shed more pounds than a fast run, according to a small study in Greece. In the three-month study, 14 women who exercised at a moderate pace lost more weight than the women who exercised more vigorously. The researchers suggest striving for a combination of moderate and vigorous exercise — with your doctor's approval — for the most benefits. When you exercise strenuously, you rev up your metabolism, and you'll continue to burn more calories long after you stop exercising.

If you are thinking about buying an exercise machine, consider this — the best choice for burning calories is a treadmill. Wear your walking shoes when you shop for a treadmill so you can try it out in the store. Make sure the controls and handrails are located comfortably and the belt fits your stride. You can probably get along fine with a less durable — and less expensive — treadmill if you are only using it for walking. Hop on for 10 minutes at a time about four times a day for the best results.

Resistance, or strength, training is a great way to replace fat with muscle. You can do these exercises at home with equipment ranging from simple household items to sophisticated gear from a sporting goods store. You can also join a health club or fitness center for a wider range of equipment and trainers to help you decide the exact exercises you need.

People age 55 and older account for about 25 percent of all gym and health club memberships, and many programs are designed for middle-age and older adults. One program, available to people who have reached age 65, is the SilverSneakers Fitness Program. Benefits include a free membership at a participating fitness center, as well as exercise classes geared for seniors. Certain Medicare Advantage plans offer the program at no extra cost. For more information, call 866-584-7389 toll free or visit *www.silversneakers.com* on the Internet.

This gym alternative keeps your waist trim

Have you ever felt so overwhelmed at the gym that you didn't want to go back? If so, gardening may be the perfect choice for you. It's easy to weave into your daily routine and is a good way to transition into a more active lifestyle.

When you garden, you get a workout all over. And that helps you control your weight. A study in the *American Journal of Public Health* found that people who worked in their community garden had a significantly lower body mass index than their neighbors who didn't.

That may not come as a surprise since gardening is an excellent way to burn calories. Expect to use up 200 to 400 calories every hour you're gardening.

Natural alternatives to common drugs

Herb	May replace*	What it does	May interact with
aloe	Metamucil	Relieves constipation	hypoglycemic drugs, insulin
black cohosh	hormone-replacement therapy (HRT) drugs	Eases menopausal symptoms	birth control pills, tamoxifen
garlic	aspirin, ibuprofen	Reduces pain and inflammation of rheumatoid arthritis	saquinavir, warfarin and other anticoagulants, antiplatelet drugs, NSAIDs, fish oil
	cholesterol-lowering drugs	Lowers cholesterol, stops blood from clumping, and slows the stiffening of arteries	
ginger	Dramamine	Relieves motion sickness, including dizziness, nausea, and vomiting	anticoagulants, NSAIDs, insulin
peppermint	Milk of Magnesia	Relieves upset stomach	antacids, cyclosporine, felodipine, simvastatin
	Nyquil	Relieves nighttime cold symptoms and cough	
	Pamprin	Acts as a muscle relaxant to relieve cramps	

Natural alternatives to common drugs

Herb	May replace*	What it does	May interact with
peppermint oil	Tylenol Vicks VapoRub Bengay	Relieves headaches Reduces congestion Relieves muscle pain	antacids, cyclosporine, felodipine, simvastatin
red clover	Proscar (finasteride)	May relieve some symptoms of benign prostatic hyperplasia (BPH)	anticoagulants, birth control pills, NSAIDs
saw palmetto	Proscar (finasteride)	Increases urine flow while decreasing urination frequency. May reduce prostate size in BPH	testosterone (Androderm), HRT, anticoagulants, NSAIDs
St. John's wort	antidepressants	May relieve mild depression	antidepressants, cyclosporine, protease inhibitors, birth control pills, warfarin, anesthetics, statins
valerian	Ambien, Valium	Helps relieve anxiety and tension while providing a good night's sleep	antidepressants, alcohol

Do not stop taking any prescription drugs without talking to your doctor first.

Index

and high blood pressure 200
caution 247
for gout 173
for osteoarthritis 247-248
for shingles 309
for sinusitis 317
interactions, drug 299

O

Oatmeal
for rosacea 304
bath 309
for cancer prevention 60
Obstructive sleep apnea.
See Sleep apnea
Ocular rosacea 303-304.
See Also Rosacea
Office of Dietary Supplements 347
Olive oil
and gallstones 145
for cancer prevention 61
for constipation 105-106
for psoriasis 273-274
Omega-3 fatty acids
and Alzheimer's disease 12
and flaxseed 206
and stroke 338
for asthma 30
for depression 112
for heart disease 187-188
for high blood pressure 196
for IBD 220
for psoriasis 272
for rheumatoid arthritis 291-292
for stress relief 24
Oral allergy syndrome 7
Orange juice
and Alzheimer's disease 12
and calcium 267
and GERD 151
and iron absorption 285
and stroke 338

for cataracts 85
for rheumatoid arthritis 292
Osteoarthritis 247-256, 288
Osteoporosis 258-268
Outpatient surgery 20

P

Partnership for Prescription
Assistance (PPA) 99
Patient Assistance Programs
(PAPs) 99
Patient Services, Inc, copay
assistance 100
Peppermint
and GERD 152
for headaches 359
for upset stomach 358
oil 253-255
tea 320
Periodic limb movement disorder
(PLMD) 287-288
Periodontitis. *See* Gingivitis;
Gum disease
PET scan 15
Pets 117, 187, 230
Pharmacy discounts 100
Phobias 24
Physical therapy, self-care 37-38,
42-43
Pill splitting 81
Pistachios, and heart disease 189-190
Planks 43-44
Plant-based diet 294
Plants, indoor 2
Plums, dried, for osteoporosis
262-263
Pollution, outdoor, and stroke 340
Pomegranate juice, for cancer
prevention 59-60
Portion control, and weight gain
348-349

Tools, adaptive 172-173
Toothbrushes 166
Toxins, environmental 78-80
Transient ischemic attack (TIA)
    334. *See Also* Stroke
Tryptophan 234
Turmeric. *See Also* Curcumin
    and gallstones 143
    for cancer prevention 60
    for cataracts 85-86
    for depression 116-117
    for flu 137
    for GERD 154-155
    for IBD 214
    for psoriasis 273
    for rheumatoid arthritis 291

U

U.S. Pharmacopeia seal 265
Ulcerative colitis (UC) 214-220
Ultraviolet (UV) rays, cataracts
    and 84
Undergarments, for
    incontinence 228
Urinary incontinence (UI).
    See Incontinence
Urinary tract infections (UTIs)
    341-346
Urogynecologist, for
    incontinence 226
Urologist, for incontinence 226
USDA Food Pyramid 163

V

Vaccines
    chickenpox 308
    flu 132-134, 139, 185
    pneumonia 133, 185
    shingles 311

Vagus nerve stimulation, for
    depression 111
Valerian 23, 359
Varicella-zoster virus 307
Vegetarian diet 145, 352-353. *See Also*
    Plant-based diet
Vision problems
    age-related macular degeneration
        (AMD) 91
    and dementia 89
    and turmeric 85-86
    Knight's Templar Eye
        Foundation 90
    Mission Cataract USA 90
    tips for 89
VitaCost 215
Vitamin A
    for allergies 8
    for asthma 29-30
    for osteoporosis 258-259
    for sinusitis 319
Vitamin B12 258
Vitamin C
    and cancer therapy 72-73
    and colds 97-98
    and gallstones 144
    and IBD 220
    and Raynaud's syndrome 279
    and rheumatoid arthritis 292
    for allergies 5
    for asthma 29-30
    for BPH 53
    for gingivitis 164
    for gout 171
    for sinusitis 318
Vitamin D
    and flu 135
    and IBD 219
    and migraines 242-243
    dosage 66
    for cancer prevention 70-71
    for gingivitis 164